SOME FACTS TO LIVE BY:

- **High blood pressure can occur in thirty- to forty-five year olds—not just in the elderly.**

- **Hypertension affects calm, even-tempered people —not just tense or highstrung personalities.**

- **There are medical treatments available now that control your blood pressure with minimal side effects.**

Lower Your Blood Pressure and Live Longer takes a revolutionary approach to the detection and treatment of high blood pressure. Specialist Dr. Marvin Moser offers a simple and highly effective program that lets you take control of your own healthy future—with a regime that fits into every lifestyle.

You'll learn the basic facts about these conditions and their warning signals; the effects of smoking and alcohol in the hypertense person; pregnancy and high blood pressure; diet, exercise, and the prevention of heart disease; treatment fads and frauds; case histories; charts on medication and side effects; low-salt and low-fat dietary guidelines—*and much more!*

D0042770

ABOUT THE AUTHOR

MARVIN MOSER, M.D., is a practicing cardiologist in White Plains, New York. He is clinical professor of medicine at the Yale University School of Medicine, and the senior medical consultant to the National High Blood Pressure Education Program of the National Heart, Lung, and Blood Institute. He is also emeritus chief of the cardiology section at the White Plains, New York, Hospital Medical Center, and a fellow of the Council for High Blood Pressure Research of the American Heart Association. Dr. Moser has been actively involved in hypertension research for over thirty years, and has authored three medical texts and over three hundred scientific papers in the field of cardiology and hypertension. In 1985 he received the National High Blood Pressure Education Program Award for outstanding contributions in the treatment of hypertension. Dr. Moser lives in Westchester County, New York.

LOWER YOUR BLOOD PRESSURE AND LIVE LONGER

MARVIN MOSER, M.D.

BERKLEY BOOKS, NEW YORK

This Berkley book contains the complete
text of the original hardcover edition.

LOWER YOUR BLOOD PRESSURE AND LIVE LONGER

A Berkley Book / published by arrangement with
Villard Books

PRINTING HISTORY
Villard edition / May 1989
Published simultaneously in Canada by
Random House of Canada Limited, Toronto
Berkley edition / March 1991

ISBN: 0-425-12675-7

A BERKLEY BOOK ® TM 757,375
Berkley Books are published by The Berkley Publishing Group,
200 Madison Avenue, New York, New York 10016.
The name "Berkley" and the "B" logo
are trademarks belonging to Berkley Publishing Corporation.

To my wife, Joy

ACKNOWLEDGMENTS

This book was written in close collaboration with Mrs. Genell Subak-Sharpe. Her suggestions, revisions, and editing were major contributions to this book. My thanks to Emily Fraenkel and Laura Rosenfield who assisted in the typing and editing process. Mrs. Adrienne Cramer has been a research associate of mine for more than twenty years, and her contributions, not only to this book, but to my research efforts through the years, have been invaluable. I am also grateful to Ms. Diane Reverand, executive editor at Villard Books, for her helpful suggestions and critique of the manuscript. Roy and Ted Benjamin of the Benjamin Company, who published the patient education booklet "High Blood Pressure and What You Can Do About It," should be thanked for their help in distributing this booklet over the past ten years.

I would like to acknowledge the major contributions to hypertension control in the United States of Mrs. Mary Lasker and Mrs. Alice Fordyce of the Lasker Foundation. Their efforts led to increased research and treatment support for state and local hypertension treatment programs. Dr. Michael DeBakey of the Baylor School of Medicine, with whom I served on the National Citizens Committee for the Treatment of High Blood Pressure, has also contributed significantly to the hypertension control effort in the United States. Dr. Claude Lenfant, Director of the National Heart, Lung, and Blood Institute of the National Institutes of Health, Bethesda, Maryland, should be cited for his considerable ongoing support of research in heart disease and hypertension. Dr. Edward Rocella, Coordinator of the National High Blood Pressure Education Program, deserves a special note of commendation for his continuing efforts to reduce strokes and heart disease by promoting educational efforts to reduce heart disease risk factors. I have had the pleasure of being the Senior Consultant to this national program for over fifteen years. My gratitude to several friends and colleagues of long standing—Dr. Irvine Page, who for many years was head of the Department of Hypertension Research of the Cleveland Clinic and is one of the original thinkers and researchers in the field of hypertension, provides a role model for physicians who seek answers to our yet unsolved problems. Drs. Raymond Gifford and Harriet Dustan who also did most of their research work in hypertension at the Cleveland Clinic and who have provided leadership in the field for many years. Dr. Edward Freis, who received the Albert Lasker Award for his pioneering efforts in demonstrating that the lowering of blood pressure prevented strokes and heart failure; I am grateful to him for his guidance (as long ago as 1951) in Washington when I was involved in hypertension research at the Walter Reed Army Medical Center. And Dr. William Dock, who is now in Paris and remains one of the Renaissance Men in medicine; He taught me the importance of the risk factor concept in medicine in 1947, at a time when most physicians were unaware or disinterested in preventive cardiology.

I would also like to acknowledge my gratitude to all the members of the National High Blood Pressure Coordinating Committee of the National Heart, Lung, and Blood Institute, with whom I have worked closely over the past fifteen years, and to the many organizations such as the American Heart Association and the American

College of Cardiology who have helped shape my ideas and thoughts about the treatment and control of major public health problems. And to my colleagues, from whom I have learned so much, and the students at the Albert Einstein College of Medicine, the New York Medical College and at the Yale University School of Medicine, with whom I have interacted over the past thirty years. And finally, to the patients whom I have treated over the years and who have helped me to retain some of the humanity and art of medicine that is rapidly being lost in a profession that is increasingly being driven by technology and entrepreneurism.

CONTENTS

Acknowledgments   vii
Introduction   xiii
1. *What Is High Blood Pressure?*   1
2. *Diagnosing High Blood Pressure*   18
3. *The Effects of High Blood Pressure*   44
4. *Who Should Treat Your High Blood Pressure?*   70
5. *The Role of Diet*   81
6. *The Role of Exercise*   116
7. *Drugs to Lower Blood Pressure*   132
8. *Biofeedback, Relaxation, and Other Nondrug Therapies*   178
9. *What Is Your Role in Treatment?*   185
10. *What About Smoking?*   197
11. *What About Alcohol?*   210
12. *The Cholesterol Question*   221
13. *Special Problems of Hypertension in Women*   238
14. *Hypertension in Children*   254
15. *Hypertension in the Elderly*   266
16. *Putting It All in Perspective*   278
Glossary   283
Epilogue   289

INTRODUCTION

This book brings good news for the more than fifty to sixty million Americans who have high blood pressure or other risk factors of heart disease. Unfortunately we live in an era where good news is equated with "no news." Much of what you'll read here has never made front-page headlines or had television coverage. What you'll learn on the following pages not only can help you live longer but will also help relieve your concerns about having high blood pressure or developing such complications as heart disease, stroke, or kidney disease. If you follow some of the suggestions in this book, you may also be able to save thousands of dollars in unnecessary medical tests and procedures, some of which are frightening, uncomfortable, and even dangerous, and to protect yourself, at least partially, from a medical care system that increasingly serves technologists rather than patients.

The good news hit home at the April 1987 National High Blood Pressure Program meeting. Dr. Claude Lenfant, director of the National Heart, Lung and Blood Institute, announced that since 1972 the death rate from strokes had fallen an incredible 50.2 percent and that deaths from heart attacks had dropped by more than 35 percent. As I listened to this progress report, I recalled the gloomy predictions of the 1950's, 1960's, and early 1970's. At that time heart attacks claimed more than a million lives a year, and strokes about three hundred thousand. Experts had warned that because of our aging population, we could expect even higher death rates in the coming decades. After all, the older we get, the more heart and blood vessel disease we are supposed to have. But something remarkable had happened. Instead of rising, the death toll from two of our most relentless serious diseases had been cut by one third to one half. It is important to establish the reasons for this dramatic decrease in death rates from heart disease, which remains the leading cause of death in the United States, and from stroke, the third leading cause of death.

In my opinion, the most important reason for this decline is the improved detection and treatment of high blood pressure during the last fifteen to twenty years. This is especially true for the reduction of strokes and stroke deaths. Approximately 75 to 80 percent of strokes occur in people with high blood pressure. Better treatment has obviously made a difference. Of course, Americans, especially middle-aged men, are smoking less. All of us are eating fewer fatty foods and are exercising more. These life-style changes, in addition to better blood pressure control and technological advances in surgery, probably play a role in the declining death rates from heart disease.

Members of the press listened to Dr. Lenfant's announcement at this meeting, but what little they reported the next day was buried. I suspect that had the institute announced a 1 percent *rise* in stroke deaths or that the use of one of the many medications used in the treatment of high blood pressure had caused a few cases of hepatitis, the news would have made page one and prime-time television. Yes, good news unfortunately is often equated with no news. Still, lack of attention by the press does not alter the happy facts for the millions of Americans with high blood pressure.

Despite our remarkable advances in recent years, there are still people who believe that it does little good to treat high blood pressure, especially when it is not very severe. Their attitude harks back fifty years or so and is summed up in the following quote from a 1931 *British Medical Journal:* "The greatest danger to a man with high blood pressure lies in its discovery because then some fool is certain to try and reduce it."

To give you an idea of how far we have come from the days when many physicians believed that having high blood pressure might actually be good for you, I want to review the medical history of President Franklin Delano Roosevelt and compare his treatment and its unhappy outcome with what would have happened today. In 1935, when Mr. Roosevelt was fifty-three years old, he had a normal blood pressure of 136/78. By 1937 it was 162/98. Despite the fact that he had no symptoms or signs of damage to his heart, kidneys, or other organs, he probably would have been treated even in the 1960's, and his blood pressure would have been reduced to normal (below 140/90).

In 1937 there were no effective drugs or other treatments for high blood pressure. Roosevelt remained untreated, and the disease was left to progress on a relentless course. By 1940 his blood pressure was 178/98, and in 1941, at the beginning of World War II, it was 188/105. He still did not experience any specific symptoms, and he appeared to be successfully performing his demanding presidential duties during one of the nation's most difficult periods. By 1944, when his blood pressure reached 188/110, there was evidence of heart enlargement. Roosevelt's doctors put him on a low-fat diet and prescribed phenobarbital, a mild sedative, along with massages. These were standard treatments for that time, but doctors knew they were largely ineffective. Many really didn't believe that lowering blood pressure was actually helpful.

In late 1944, with the war effort at its height, the President began to suffer from heart failure and headaches. He could not lie flat in bed without experiencing shortness of breath because of the accumulation of fluid in his lungs. So night after night he sat up in a chair, sleeping only three or four hours. The lack of sleep, as much as his worsening medical condition, may have accounted for his sickly, wan appearance in the last months of his life and for the fact that some observers questioned his effectiveness. By early 1945 his blood pressure was extremely high, ranging between 180/110 and 230/125–130. On April 12, 1945, at the young age of sixty-three, he suffered a massive stroke and died within an hour.

Mr. Roosevelt's blood pressure was only moderately elevated until near the end of his life. Of course, not all people with mild hypertension progress and die of heart failure or stroke within five to ten years after the discovery of elevated blood pressure, but prior to the 1950's many did. Today, with the wide array of highly effective treatments to lower blood pressure, the large majority of patients like Mr. Roosevelt remain healthy and productive, with normal life-spans.

Unfortunately we still see people who are told that their blood pressure is only "slightly high," that they are "just nervous," or that their elevated blood pressure is the result of the white coat syndrome—meaning it is high in the presence of a doctor but normal at other times. Many of these individuals end up later with evidence of heart or kidney disease that could have been prevented by earlier treatment.

An example of what can happen is illustrated in the case history of a lawyer patient of mine. I first saw him more than thirty years ago in 1955. He had been told for many years that he just had "slightly high blood pressure," which was attributed to "nervousness." He was not experiencing any symptoms and was carrying on a demanding law practice. His physician had decided he did not need any treatment.

The patient went about his business, not realizing that he had a potentially serious problem. He had not had his blood pressure taken for three years prior to his coming to me at the age of forty-two for an insurance examination. He still had no symptoms; but his blood pressure was 220/130, and there was evidence of heart enlargement despite his *relatively* young age. At the time his prognosis was not particularly good. People with this level of blood pressure and these findings usually do not live for more than three to five years if the pressure is left untreated. Sadly his health problems were not entirely his fault. His doctor should have at least insisted on routine follow-up exams and should have detected the rising blood pressure.

Nevertheless, he was lucky. Treatment was undertaken, blood pressure controlled, and he lived for another twenty-eight years. (At the age of seventy he died of a ruptured aneurysm—a burst blood vessel, which may very well have been weakened years before when his pressure was high.) Some patients are not as fortunate as he. I can relate numerous similar reports that did not have such a satisfactory outcome. What is particularly sad is the fact that high blood pressure is a disease that is easy to detect and can be treated effectively.

If controlling high blood pressure is so straightforward, why am I writing this book? Isn't there lots of other information available to the public about high blood pressure? There are several reasons to justify my undertaking. First and foremost, I want to demystify this disease, which is medically referred to as hypertension.

Although we can control high blood pressure, we still do not know the cause of hypertension or how to cure it permanently in more than 90 percent of cases, but we can treat it successfully *without* knowing all about its causes. And we can treat it simply without discomfort or great expense to the patient.

Another reason for this book is that I have always believed that patients should be informed about their illnesses and about how their doctors plan to treat them. Yes, we physicians all give lip service to patient education, yet look around the next time you visit your doctor to see if there is any readable, up-to-date literature available on hypertension. After all, hypertension is the most frequent reason that adults see their physicians. And how much informative material is there in the waiting room or treatment rooms about diabetes, heart disease, or other common diseases? Not much. This book grew out of a pamphlet entitled *High Blood Pressure and What You Can Do About It* that I have been using for patient education for more than twenty-five years. This pamphlet has also been distributed by the National Heart, Lung and Blood Institute's National High Blood Pressure Education Program for the last seven to ten years. All of us will admit that reading material isn't the only way to help someone understand a medical problem, but today physicians are often too busy to "start from scratch" and explain everything. Thus, reading informative materials will help supplement the doctor's message.

As with so many chronic diseases, there are lots of myths relating to hypertension and dozens of remedies being advocated. Some of these may have merit, but often they are accepted and publicized without sufficient proof of their effectiveness. All of us would like to control our own destinies, including taking charge of our health. We can do this in many instances, but we must remember that it is not always possible. We may have to depend on medications and on specific medical care for help. Unfortunately, in today's world of defensive, technologically oriented medicine, common sense in medical care is too often overlooked and the "help" becomes a complex maze. Far too many patients fall victim to a kind of medical overkill. They end up having too many tests, taking unnecessarily expensive new drugs when older ones may work just as well, and turning their lives upside down in the mistaken belief that this is "good or quality medical care."

Good medical care, in many instances, may be *less* medical care. Too many of today's physicians have abdicated the traditional humanistic approach and rely on technology rather than on their own good judgment and experience. Given today's legal climate, far too many doctors are practicing defensive medicine, ordering every test and procedure in the book just in case they later find themselves defending their treatments in court. As a result, we *all* suffer, and if the present trends continue unchecked, we may well find ourselves with the world's most expensive but not necessarily best health care system.

Actually the large majority of people with mild to moderate high blood pressure (hypertension) can be treated with a relatively simple regimen without a major change in life-style. They don't need to turn their households into diet kitchens in an effort to lower their blood pressure or prevent heart disease. They don't have to camp out at their doctors' office, become exercise fanatics, or spend thousands of dollars on a battery of complicated tests that often will not provide any information that will change either their treatments or their futures. Of course, there are cases in which modern technology must be used for a specific diagnosis or treatment, but these cases are not the rule.

This book is intended to give you the facts about the detection, treatment, and possible prevention of high blood pressure and other risk factors for heart disease and to help you become an informed partner in making important decisions regarding your own health care. It should help you determine if a particular test or treatment is justified and which factors have been proved to be important in preventing heart disease and stroke. While the technology of modern medicine has helped save lives, it is being overused in my opinion. Science and technology are not substitutes for rationality, common sense, and correct information. With a proper balance, you can control your high blood pressure and other risk factors for heart disease and lead a long, productive life free from needless health fears. I believe that this book will help you achieve that balance.

1

WHAT IS
HIGH BLOOD PRESSURE?

More than forty million adult Americans have high blood pressure—or hypertension, to use its medical name—making it our most common chronic illness. Despite tremendous advances in both the detection and the treatment of hypertension, there are still many people, perhaps several million, who are unaware that they have high blood pressure. This is understandable because unlike many other diseases, hypertension can exist and progress for decades without producing any symptoms. Hypertension is directly or indirectly responsible for several hundred thousand deaths in this country each year. It is a major cause of strokes and one of three major risk factors for heart attacks—our number one cause of death. About 20 to 25 percent of patients who have kidney failure and are on dialysis programs in the United States started out with "just a little high blood pressure" ten, fifteen, or twenty years before their kidneys stopped working properly.

The statistics are grim. Yet for the large majority of patients, high blood pressure is easy to diagnose, and there is now a wide array of effective treatments that almost always can bring it under control. And with adequate control the potentially lethal effects of hypertension can be avoided. In short, hypertension should no longer be considered a frightening disease. Obviously it cannot be taken lightly, but an informed patient with high blood pressure who follows a simple but structured regimen can lead a normal, productive, and long life.

How the Circulatory System Works

Blood pressure, as the term implies, is the amount of force exerted against the artery walls as blood flows through the body. Exactly how the body regulates blood pressure is not completely understood, but we do know that many different organs—principally, the heart, the kidneys, the brain, and the blood vessels themselves—are involved. The human circulatory system is a marvel. Each one of us has about 60,000 miles of blood vessels, ranging in size from about 0.8 to 0.0004 of an inch in diameter. Blood traveling through this intricate network of vessels carries oxygen and other life-sustaining nutrients to every cell of the body and also picks up waste material for elimination through the kidneys or lungs.

The average adult has about eleven pints of blood, which constantly circulates through the body. Every minute the heart beats an average of sixty to seventy times at rest, and with each beat, two or three ounces of blood are pumped from the heart's left ventricle or major pumping chamber into the aorta, the body's largest artery. The aorta, which carries blood with a high content of oxygen, branches off into smaller blood vessels or tubes called arteries, which in turn branch off into even smaller arterioles—the body's tiniest arteries. The aorta is like the main trunk of a tree, the arteries are like the larger branches, and the arterioles are like small branches or twigs. The arterioles branch into capillaries, and from these microscopic vessels, all of the body's cells—in the arms, legs, brain, lungs, and elsewhere—exchange carbon dioxide and other waste material for fresh oxygen and other nutrients that are carried to them in the blood. The "used" blood, high in carbon dioxide, then passes from the capillaries into thinner but larger vessels called venules, which branch into larger veins. Eventually the oxygen-depleted blood ends up back in the *right* side of the heart and is pumped into the lungs to get a fresh supply of oxygen and to begin anew its trip through the body. It's a remarkable system that is efficient enough to adapt constantly to our needs. When we exercise, for example, the whole process speeds up; the heart beats 100 to 125 or more times a minute, and the amount of blood pumped out may double or triple. When we have a large meal, blood vessels in the abdomen dilate and supply more blood to our stomachs or intestinal tracts so that food can be more easily digested. All this requires a "head of pressure" in our blood vessels to keep the blood moving forward. An excessive drop in pressure will be felt almost immediately with symptoms or findings depending on the system affected. For example, if the brain doesn't get enough blood, we faint. If too little blood gets to the kidneys over a prolonged period of time, they function less effectively; urine output drops and waste products build up in the blood. If we go swimming thirty to forty-five minutes after a large meal, and extra blood is required by our arms and legs, less blood is made available for digesting food, and we may experience stomach cramps. The factors that regulate blood flow to our vital organs are extremely fine-tuned.

High blood pressure occurs when too much force or pressure is exerted against the walls of the arteries. To visualize how the circulatory system works, imagine that it is modeled after a plumbing system. The heart's action is comparable to a faucet: Open a faucet and water flows from it, similar to what happens when the heart beats and pumps blood into the aorta or the arteries to the lungs. When the faucet is closed, water ceases to flow, comparable to what happens when the heart rests between beats.

The arteries may be likened to the water pipes or tubes of a plumbing system, with the arterioles, which contain large amounts of smooth muscle tissue that is capable of squeezing down or opening wider, functioning like a nozzle. When a nozzle is open, water flows freely through it. Similarly, when the arterioles' tiny controlling muscles are relaxed, they are fully open or dilated, permitting a free flow of blood into the next smallest group of blood vessels. But when the muscles tighten, the arterioles become constricted, or narrowed, similar to what happens when you close down a nozzle. Thus, by widening or narrowing, these tiny vessels help control blood pressure. For example, when blood is pumped into constricted or narrowed arterioles, there is a buildup of pressure against the walls, just as there is a buildup of water pressure against the sides of a hose if you turn on a faucet but keep the nozzle partially or totally closed. Of course, the body's circulation is a closed system (blood doesn't leak out anywhere), in which the blood must keep moving, even if the arterioles are narrowed or constricted. If they remain constricted, the system responds, for example, by making the heart work harder to increase the blood pressure and force the blood forward. High blood pressure, or hypertension, then occurs.

Contrary to popular belief, blood pressure does not remain constant but fluctuates according to body demands and activities. In fact, it is not unusual for blood pressure to vary by as much as 20 or 30 points in a day. It rises during periods when extra blood is needed, such as when you exercise. It also rises when you are tense or angry; this is a part of the body's fight-or-flight response. It is usually lower during sleep or inactivity. It is of interest to note that blood pressure levels are the highest in the early-morning hours just before and as we awaken, say from 6:00 to 8:00 A.M. This probably is related to the stirring of the nervous system, which has been "asleep" for several or more hours. Pressure generally stays at these levels throughout the day, until about 10:00 P.M. to midnight, when they begin to fall. From about 1:00 to 4:00 A.M. blood pressures are at their lowest.

The force that moves blood through the circulatory system originates in the heart, but many other organs and control mechanisms help maintain and monitor blood pressure. These controls can be compared with sophisticated thermostats that can sense minute changes and make necessary adjustments to ensure that the right amount of blood is flowing through the body to the right places. When you stand up suddenly, the body makes an almost instantaneous adjustment in blood pressure to ensure that a decrease in the amount of blood reaching the brain does not occur. Signals are sent out to increase the rate of the heartbeat and to narrow down or constrict the little arteries. Sometimes there is a slight delay in the control system, and temporary dizziness or light-headedness may be noted. In extreme cases fainting may occur. This may be noted after you have had a heavy meal or several alcoholic drinks or after you have been sitting in the sun or standing for a long time in a hot room. Alcohol or heat can cause the blood vessels in muscles and the skin to dilate. After a heavy meal too much blood may be diverted to the digestive system, reducing the amount that gets up to the brain. Prolonged standing can result in a pooling of blood in the legs. In such instances fainting is nature's way of redistributing the blood flow; it causes us to "get flat" so that the blood can more easily be pumped to our heads.

In such circumstances fainting usually is not dangerous, although there is a hazard of injury while falling, and after fainting, a person may feel tired. In this era of malpractice suits, however, fainting may carry a new hazard. I was summoned on the double during a recent hospital benefit party to examine a woman in her sixties who had fainted. She was surrounded by paramedics who were getting her ready to be transported to the hospital for observation. This is the usual procedure—frequently because it is necessary, but just as often to protect against the claim that everything that could have been done wasn't. In this instance no one had taken the trouble to find out that she had eaten very little, had had a few cocktails, and had been standing still for about an hour in a hot, crowded room. This is the perfect setup for fainting: Blood had pooled in her legs and abdomen, and not enough was reaching her brain. It wasn't easy to convince the medics that all would be well if we just let her sit quietly and get a second wind. This case illustrates a good lesson in commonsense medicine. If someone faints under these circumstances *and has no other symptoms,* don't panic. Help the person get to a cool spot to rest for a few minutes. Lying down with a pillow under the legs and feet will increase blood flow to the brain. Chances are, in a few minutes the person will fully recover. This is how I treated the woman described above, sparing her a trip to the hospital, an overnight stay for observation, and a good deal of worry and anxiety for her and her family.

Of course, blood does not flow in a steady stream, like water from an open faucet. It moves in spurts that correspond to the heart's beat. With each beat there is a surge in blood flow as the heart's pumping chamber ejects a new spurt of blood into the circulation. The pressure in the artery that results from this surge is called the systolic pressure; it is the maximum force of blood against the artery walls. In a normal blood pressure reading of 120/80, the higher or upper number represents the systolic pressure. The force in the artery decreases when the heart rests between beats; the pressure that remains is called the resting or diastolic pressure and is represented by the lower number in the reading. During this period, when pressure is at its lowest, blood enters the capillaries and then begins the return journey to the heart. Blood is constantly moving in wavelike surges through the entire circulatory system.

How Blood Pressure Is Measured

The discovery of blood pressure and how to measure it provides a fascinating glimpse into the history of medicine. Although ancient physicians had studied anatomy and mapped out the body's blood vessels, it was not until 1628 that William Harvey, the pioneering English court doctor, discovered that blood actually circulates or moves through the body. Even though many early physicians and scientists, including Galileo, had measured and studied pulsebeats, they had not associated them with the heart and circulation. Dr. Harvey changed this with the publication of his monograph *De Motu Cordis et Sanguinis in Animalibus,* ("On the Motion of the Heart and Blood in Animals") in which he described the heart's role in maintaining the circulation of blood through the body.

It took another hundred years before blood pressure was actually measured. That landmark discovery did not come from a physician; instead, it was made by Stephen Hales, an English clergyman who used his horse for an experiment. With the animal tied down in a lying position, the Reverand Hales inserted a hollow needle into one of the horse's arteries. The needle was connected to a flexible tube, which in turn was attached to a long glass tube with water in it. He calculated the pressure in the artery by measuring how high the water rose in the tube. During a heartbeat the water rose to a height of eight feet three inches, and between heartbeats it dropped dramatically. We now know that these surges and falls represented the systolic and diastolic pressures. The Reverend Hales's discovery obviously was important, but hardly suitable for routine medical examinations. He had had to puncture an artery, and the measuring apparatus was cumbersome, to say the least. An eight-foot tube of water is certainly not a practical way to measure pressure. Eventually researchers discovered that blood pressure could be measured externally, without inserting a needle into an artery, and that substances other than water could be used. In 1896 Scipione Riva-Rocci, an Italian physician, invented the portable blood pressure machine whose basic design is still used today. This machine, called a sphygmomanometer (pronounced sfig-moe-man-OM-a-ter), consists of an inflatable rubber cuff and an air pump. A column of mercury is used instead of water. (Mercury is used because it is much heavier than water and the pressure in the artery generated by the heartbeat will push the mercury column up to only a fraction of the level that it pushes water.) Blood pressure readings are expressed in millimeters (mm) of mercury (Hg), abbreviated as mmHg. Thus, doctors will record pressure as 120/80 mmHg with 120 the systolic or pumping pressure and 80 the diastolic or resting pressure.

The cuff is wrapped around an arm (or a leg in rare instances), and air is pumped into it. The idea is to determine how much pressure is needed to stop the flow of blood through the major artery of the arm or leg. The diaphragm of a stethoscope is placed over the artery below the cuff (at the inner side of the bend in the arm at the elbow). As air is pumped into the cuff and it tightens around the arm, the air pressure will drive up the column of mercury. After the cuff has been tightened, the doctor will listen for sounds through the stethoscope and keep pumping air until sounds stop. This means that blood flow in the artery beyond the cuff has been stopped. The air is then gradually released, and the cuff is loosened. When a thumping sound is heard, it indicates that blood is beginning to spurt back into the artery. The height of the mercury when the first thump is heard represents the systolic or pumping pressure. The cuff is further loosened by releasing more air and allowing the artery to open fully; sounds heard through the stethoscope gradually disappear. The height of the mercury when these thumping sounds cease represents the diastolic or resting blood pressure.

This sounds complicated, but the entire process takes less than a minute. There also are blood pressure machines that have thin metal bellows that cause a needle to move on a dial. These are called aneroid (or air) blood pressure recorders; they are usually accurate and not subject to too many problems. These are the most commonly used devices for home blood pressure taking. Some blood pressure devices use electronic sensors and a digital printout on a small screen. These instruments may be very sensitive and can give falsely high readings since any motion in the hand or arm (clenching a fist or even moving fingers) may trigger the sensor. When these instruments are used and a high reading that doesn't seem right is recorded, the procedure should be repeated. For example, if your blood pressures are usually about 140–150/90 mmHg and if, using an electronic home blood pressure machine, you record a level of 200/110 mmHg, chances are it's an error. Unfortunately many people are unaware of the sensitivity of these types of instruments and become alarmed when high readings are noted. If repeated unusual readings are obtained, you should see your doctor. It's a good idea to take along your blood pressure machine so that it, too, can be checked. The problem may be in the machine or your technique, not your actual blood pressure.

The home blood pressure machines that are electronic are highly automated, eliminating the need for a stethoscope. This may be an advantage in a case where a person is hard-of-hearing or lives alone and cannot manage to pump up the cuff and also handle a stethoscope, but as noted, there may be disadvantages to their use. All the different blood pressure recording devices are useful under certain conditions, but the old-fashioned cuff and column of mercury is still considered the most accurate and is generally preferred by doctors. Most physicians also find the aneroid instrument with a needle on a dial acceptable.

In rare instances, such as in a hospital critical care unit, a doctor may wish to monitor blood pressure directly by inserting into an artery a very fine needle attached to electronic sensing devices and recorders. This gives a precise blood pressure measurement at any given moment, but this kind of monitoring is very rarely needed and, in my opinion, is used too frequently. Remember, whenever a needle is inserted into a blood vessel and left in place, the possibility of a clot or an infection increases. Blood pressure monitoring with a needle in an artery should be necessary only during complicated surgery (such as a coronary bypass operation) or when someone is in shock and pressures are difficult to take in the usual ways.

In recent years a number of doctors have begun recommending continuous blood pressure monitoring. In this examination a person wears a portable computerized blood pressure monitor as he or she goes about routine activities. This test is expensive, costing an average of between two hundred and three hundred dollars for a twenty-four-hour recording. It has a limited place in establishing a diagnosis or in a treatment regimen and is rarely needed. The technology *is* exciting, and like many other new machines, it has captured the attention of the media before its value to the patient has been proved. During the past year I have had more than twenty requests to do this test from patients who heard about it on a television health news program or read about it in newspapers. No one told them that 20 to 30 percent of the tracings are unreadable. Even more important, we physicians have no scientific information about the technique's long-term value in treatment programs. This is a prime example of how technology is being overused and abused in modern medicine. (See Chapter 3 for a more detailed discussion.)

How High Is Too High?

There is a wide range of so-called normal blood pressures, and some doctors still disagree on where normal ends and hypertension, or high blood pressure, begins. A baby's blood pressure may be as low as 70/50; for children and adolescents, readings of less than 120/80 are normal. Throughout adulthood an average of 120/80 is regarded as ideal, although blood pressures of up to 140/90 are still considered in the normal range. If both the upper and lower readings are consistently above these numbers, then a diagnosis of hypertension is justified.

In the diagnosis of high blood pressure both the upper (the systolic) and the lower (or diastolic) numbers are important. For many years physicians and lay people alike were told that the lower reading was more important as an indicator of future problems. We now know that this is just another one of the many myths about hypertension. An elevated systolic pressure may be equally or even more predictive than the diastolic pressure of a stroke, heart attack, or heart failure. For purposes of defining hypertension, we will consider a diastolic reading of 85 to 89 high normal; 90 to 104 mild hypertension; 105 to 114 moderate, and 115 or higher severe hypertension. (See table 1:1.) Systolic readings of 140 to 159 are considered less severe hypertension; 160 to 170, moderately severe; and 180 or more, severe hypertension. In young people it is unusual to have systolic hypertension alone (readings above 160 or so) without having a high diastolic blood pressure, but in people over sixty, so-called isolated systolic hypertension with readings of 160–200/80–90 are not uncommon. Newer data suggest that many older individuals who have systolic hypertension probably had both systolic and diastolic hypertension when they were younger. The probable cause of systolic hypertension in old age is that the aorta has lost its elasticity as a result of arteriosclerosis (a medical term for hardening of the arteries). Some investigators believe that this can be prevented by early treatment of high blood pressure in younger age-groups. The terms "hypertension" and "high blood pressure," unless otherwise noted, will be used interchangeably throughout this book to define systolic and diastolic hypertension—i.e., pressures above 140/90.

About 70 percent of those diagnosed as having high blood pressure fall into the mild range (140/90 to 160/104), and most of the others have moderate hypertension (160/105 to 180/115). Today severe hypertension, which can evolve into a condition referred to as malignant hypertension, with pressures of more than 220–250/125–140 and symptoms of brain and heart damage, is very rare. This is largely due to the effective treatment of the less severe types of the disease.

TABLE 1:1

Classification of Blood Pressure*
in Adults 18 Years or Older

Range (mmHg)

DIASTOLIC

Below 85	Normal
85–90	High normal
90–104	Mild hypertension
Above 105	Moderate to severe hypertension

SYSTOLIC

Below 140	Normal
140–159	Mild elevation
Above 160	Moderate to severe elevation

EXAMPLES:

145/95:	Mild hypertension
160/105:	Moderately severe hypertension
175/115:	Severe hypertension

Adapted from the National High Blood Pressure Education Program, 1988.

*Based on the average of two or more readings on two or more occasions.

In more than 90 percent of all patients with hypertension a specific cause is never found. In fewer than one half of 1 percent, a small tumor, almost always benign, is found in one of the adrenal glands, which rest atop the kidneys. This tumor secretes a hormone that causes the body to retain salt and, consequently, to raise blood pressure. In less than one half of 1 percent of cases a different kind of tumor is noted in one or both of the adrenal glands. This secretes a great deal of adrenaline, which causes the blood vessels to narrow and constrict and thereby raises blood pressure. In about 3 to 4 percent a narrowing of an artery to one or both of the kidneys is noted. The kidney secretes an excessive amount of a substance called renin, and this eventually leads to a constriction of blood vessels, and salt retention; blood pressure goes up. Finally, in about 3 to 5 percent of patients chronic kidney disease as a result of recurrent infections or nephritis can cause hypertension. As the percentages show, all of these are uncommon. Their diagnosis will be discussed in the next chapter.

Hypertension is more common and more severe in blacks not only in industrialized societies but in rural areas such as the West Indies and the Bahamas. The reasons are unknown, but one theory holds that blacks may have a genetic tendency to conserve sodium, a component of salt. In Africa the traditional diet was very low in sodium, and salt was difficult to obtain. Over time, the kidneys of individuals with this diet became very efficient in conserving or saving sodium in order to maintain proper body chemistry. Recent studies by medical anthropologists have noted that during the 350 years of the slave trade most of the blacks died during the long, grueling boat trips to the New World. Typically they were given very little water and fed a diet of beans fried in oil.

According to this theory, the blacks who survived were those who had a genetic ability to conserve even more salt than normal. When they were later exposed to diets that were high in salt, their kidneys still tended to conserve sodium, and as a result, they retained fluid and developed high blood pressure. Whether this theory is correct is not known, but we do know that blacks in the Western Hemisphere are more efficient at retaining sodium than whites who tend to live on diets that are high in salt.

Common Myths and Facts About Hypertension

MYTH: Tense, nervous, or anxious people are likely to develop hypertension.

FACT: This myth stems partly from the medical name of the disease. People mistakenly think that "hypertension" describes a person's personality, for example, someone who is hyper or tense. In reality, "hypertension" refers to elevated pressure in the arteries, not to the personality of the individual. As stressed earlier, "hypertension" is just another term for high blood pressure. Many calm, even-tempered people have hypertension, and there also are tense, uptight, jittery types whose blood pressures are absolutely normal. It should be noted, however, that stress, anxiety, or tension can produce a temporary rise in blood pressure, and animal studies have found that prolonged stress may play a role in the development of hypertension. This has not been proved in humans.

MYTH: Older people need higher blood pressures to ensure that enough blood gets to the brain and other vital organs.

FACT: Numerous studies have found that older people with normal blood pressures of 140/90 or lower live longer and have fewer strokes, heart attacks, and heart failure than those whose pressures are even slightly elevated. As noted, even an elevation of systolic blood pressure alone increases risk. There is no proof that elevated blood pressure improves brain function in the elderly; in fact, it can have an opposite effect by increasing the chances of strokes and ministrokes—major causes of mental deterioration.

MYTH: High blood pressure is most likely to show up in old people.

FACT: Hypertension may not be diagnosed until ages sixty or older, but studies show that most cases develop between the ages of thirty and forty-five and it is also noted in younger people.

MYTH: Once you have high blood pressure, there's not much you can do to keep it from getting worse. And the treatments may be worse than the disease itself.

FACT: This is definitely false and is probably one of the most harmful of the many myths about hypertension. Recent publicity about the possible dangerous effects of medication has done a disservice to the public. Almost always the disease can be brought under control. Occasionally mild hypertension can be controlled by simple life-style changes: losing weight, cutting down on salt, moderate exercise, and so forth. Most patients, however, eventually require drug therapy. Today doctors have such a wide array of highly effective antihypertensive (blood pressure-lowering) medications that they can almost always devise a regimen that controls blood pressure with minimal side effects. *The benefit of treatment and lowering blood pressure clearly outweighs the risk.* These treatments will be described in greater detail in the following chapters.

Summing Up

• Hypertension is the leading cause of strokes and one of three major risk factors for heart attacks.

• High blood pressure occurs when too much force or pressure is exerted against the walls of the arteries.

• Blood pressure does not remain constant but fluctuates according to body demands and activities.

• In a normal blood pressure reading of 120/80 to 140/90, the higher, or upper, number represents the systolic pressure. The lower number represents the pressure in the blood vessels with the heart at rest and is called the diastolic pressure.

• Home blood pressure machines that are electronic may be less accurate than the mercury or air machines used by most doctors.

• Young people can have hypertension, too.

• Even mild or less severe hypertension (blood pressures between 140/90 and 160/105) should be treated.

2

DIAGNOSING
HIGH BLOOD PRESSURE

Not long ago an anxious woman in her mid-forties came to see me. Before I even had a chance to review her medical history, she said, "Doctor, I'm afraid I have high blood pressure." I asked what made her think so, and she replied, "My pressure is one forty-two over ninety-two, and the booklet I was given says that means I have hypertension."

Further questions revealed that she had had her blood pressure taken at a booth in an airport lobby. Her plane had been an hour late, and to kill time, she had some coffee and a cigarette in the coffee shop. Then, as she strolled through the lobby, she noticed a booth which had been set up by a physician referral service operated by a private hospital. Technicians were on hand to measure blood pressures and do five-minute cholesterol tests. There were a number of pamphlets on different ailments, each stamped with the hospital's physician referral service telephone number. All this was free, and several people were waiting for their tests.

By the time she reached the head of the line, her plane was being announced. In a rush she had her blood pressure taken—under stress and after coffee and a cigarette. It is not surprising that it was slightly elevated under these conditions, but the technicians manning the booth neglected to inform the woman of these facts. Instead, they urged her to see a doctor, and if she wanted a name, she could call the number of their referral service on the pamphlet she had been given.

I tried to reassure her that a diagnosis of hypertension could certainly not be made after a single reading under the above circumstances. As it turned out, her blood pressure was normal on readings repeated over several months. Aside from her smoking, which she has since given up, she was found to be perfectly healthy.

I relate this incident because it illustrates how all too often an inappropriate diagnosis can be made. This woman is not unique. Too many people have been rushed off to doctors to check their blood pressures and seek treatments after only one casual recording. Of course, there is nothing wrong with efforts to screen people for hypertension and detect elevated pressure at an early stage, but conditions for testing should be such that the number of falsely high readings will be minimal. In addition, someone should be available to put the blood pressure numbers in perspective. Often, however, these numbers, even when taken under inappropriate circumstances, are predictive and a follow-up is important.

Diagnostic Guidelines

Establishing the presence of high blood pressure or hypertension is relatively simple and straightforward, even though it may require several visits to the doctor's office.

Blood pressure is generally measured first with the patient seated and then again while standing, even though, in most cases, the reading taken while sitting down is adequate to make a diagnosis or guide treatment. Normally there is a slight decrease in systolic pressure and a small rise in diastolic pressure when the patient stands up. Some people, however, have overactive sympathetic nervous systems and blood pressures that increase when they stand up. The sympathetic nervous system helps control the heartbeat, the breathing system, and the rate of release of adrenaline; when adrenaline is released, both the pulse rate and blood pressures increase. Because of the excessive amount of adrenaline, people whose sympathetic nervous systems hyperreact achieve higher than normal blood pressures when they stand up suddenly. On the other hand, some people, upon standing, experience a definite fall in both systolic and diastolic pressures to low, or hypotensive, levels. This is called postural (or orthostatic) hypotension and is noted in people with diabetes and in older individuals more frequently than in the young. The presence or absence of postural hypotension may be a determining factor in the choice of a treatment program.

Guidelines for Measuring Blood Pressures

The National High Blood Pressure Education Program has established the following guidelines (with my added comments) for taking an accurate blood pressure reading.

1. The patient should be seated with the arm bare and supported at heart level. If the arm hangs down, blood pressure readings may be five to ten mmHg higher than they really are. The patient should not have smoked or ingested caffeine twenty to thirty minutes prior to measurement.

2. Measurement should begin after two to three minutes of quiet rest.

3. The appropriate cuff size should be used to ensure an accurate reading. The rubber bladder (the inflatable cuff) should encircle at least two thirds of the arm. Several sizes of cuff (e.g., child, adult, large adult) should be available. If a standard cuff is used on an obese person, for example, the readings will be higher than they should be; a large cuff is necessary.

If a person has a very thick, muscular arm, a larger cuff may also be required to get an accurate reading. I have seen at least a dozen young, athletic men referred for high blood pressure when the diagnosis proved false because of the use of small blood pressure cuffs. Several of these men were weight lifters with huge biceps. Pressures taken with a standard-size cuff were all in the high range, while the blood pressures were normal when a larger (and wider) cuff was used. This is because unusually thick muscles (or in the case of an obese person, excess fat) resist the squeezing effect of the air in the blood pressure cuff, and more pressure is required to overcome muscle or fat resistance to squeeze the artery closed. Some of the pressure recorded on the gauge may have nothing to do with actual blood pressure; instead, it is tissue resistance pressure. In this way, a falsely high blood pressure reading may be recorded. When a larger cuff is used, a wider area of the arm is compressed more evenly, less pressure is wasted in overcoming the extra tissue resistance, and a more reliable blood pressure reading is obtained.

In addition, the cuff should be wrapped securely around the arm. If it is applied loosely, the reading will also be higher than it should be.

4. Measurements should be taken with a mercury sphygmomanometer or a reliable aneroid manometer. In some cases the use of a validated electronic device is acceptable. (See Chapter 1 for descriptions of these devices.)

5. Systolic and diastolic pressures should be recorded.

6. Two or more readings (taken at different times during the same visit) should be averaged. If the first two readings differ by more than about 5 mmHg, additional readings should be obtained.

Many patients question whether blood pressures should be measured in both arms and whether or not these measurements will differ. I have done studies in which blood pressures were taken simultaneously in both arms and been found to be about the same. However, if a few minutes elapse between readings, the second will usually be somewhat lower than the first, regardless of which arm is used. (An exception might be in an older person where partial blockage of the artery leading to the left arm may result in lower readings on the left side.) In any event I take readings in both arms on the first visit and use the arm with the higher reading to guide therapy. In unusual cases the main artery to an arm (the brachial artery) may be completely blocked, making it impossible to feel a pulse or record a blood pressure on that side. Obviously the "good" arm is then used for measuring blood pressure.

The initial visit should include a careful medical history as well as a physical examination. Questions your doctor should ask—and you should be prepared to answer—include:

● Do you have a family history of high blood pressure or other cardiovascular disorders? Hypertension tends to run in families, *but even if both parents are hypertensive, it does not necessarily mean that you will develop elevated blood pressure.*

● Do you have a personal history of heart disease, cerebrovascular disorders, kidney disease, or diabetes? This is important in choosing medication.

● Have you ever been told you have high blood pressure? If so, have you undergone any kind of treatment for it? What were the results of that treatment? All too often people believe that taking medication is all that is needed for acceptable treatment, but sometimes medication is given and pressures are still not controlled. *Acceptable treatment means controlling the blood pressure.* You should know the range of your blood pressure. If pressures are in the high range, something should be done.

● Have you gained or lost significant amounts of weight? Do you consume salty foods? (Excess salt can cause the body to accumulate too much water, which may show up as a weight gain. This increased fluid volume can elevate blood pressure.)

● If you use alcohol, about how many drinks do you have a day (or week)? An intake of three or more cocktails, or more than three beers, or two to three glasses of wine a day may raise blood pressure.

● Do you smoke? Cigarette smoking is an important major risk factor for heart disease.

● What medications, including over-the-counter preparations, birth control pills, nasal sprays, antihistamines, or drugs for arthritis, are you taking? Some of these can elevate blood pressure or reduce the effectiveness of blood pressure-lowering medication.

   You may also be asked about emotional stress or other psychological or social factors that affect your overall health. Although acutely stressful situations may raise blood pressure, there is only slight evidence now that chronic stress can actually *cause* hypertension. However, if your blood pressure is high, the choice of therapy may be different if you're under stress from that recommended if your life is tranquil. Of course, you should be prepared to describe any symptoms that you have been experiencing. As you will see later, certain symptoms give clues to specific forms of hypertension, some of which are curable.

   After your doctor has taken your medical history and measured your blood pressure, perhaps two or three times, he or she will proceed to a general physical examination. In this examination particular attention is paid to signs of organ damage that may be related to high blood pressure. For example, examining the eyes is helpful because this is one of the few places where we can actually see evidence of blood vessel damage that may have resulted from high blood pressure. The eyes are the only part of the body where blood vessels can be visualized directly without an invasive procedure; by shining a light into the eyes, the doctor can see the tiny blood vessels. If pressure in these vessels has been high for some time, a thickening of the walls will be noticed. If hypertension is severe, doctors may actually see hemorrhages at the back of the eye where a small amount of blood has leaked out from the damaged vessel. This, of course, is a sign for more immediate treatment.

The neck should be carefully examined for signs of distended or enlarged veins and an enlarged thyroid gland; This could indicate either an overactive or underactive thyroid (an overactive thyroid can cause an increase in systolic blood pressure. An underactive thyroid can cause elevation of both the systolic and diastolic levels). A stethoscope will be used to listen to blood as it passes through the carotid artery, the major artery in the neck. If there is a narrowing of the vessel because of hardening of the arteries, a bruit, or hum, may be heard. Nothing specific may be done about this, but it suggests that blood vessel changes have occurred. This knowledge will help determine an appropriate course of treatment. Of course, the heart is carefully examined, with both a stethoscope and an electrocardiogram. The abdomen is felt for enlarged kidneys (a certain type of kidney enlargement can cause hypertension), and the doctor will listen for unusual sounds that may come from blood vessels in the abdomen. A bruit (a murmur or whooshing sound) near the middle of the abdomen may indicate a narrowing of one of the arteries to a kidney, and this finding could suggest a curable form of hypertension. Finally, the pulses in the legs and ankles are checked and the ankles are examined for signs of swelling.

At this stage a few laboratory tests will probably be done. A complete urinalysis, to check for evidence of kidney damage or an infection, and routine blood tests to check for diabetes, cholesterol levels, and kidney function usually provide the needed information.

Although in many cases a diagnosis of high blood pressure can be made during the initial visit, pressures are usually checked again to be sure. However, if blood pressures are very high (for example, a diastolic reading of more than 110 or 115 mmHg), or if there is clear evidence of hypertension-related damage (such as changes in the blood vessels in the eyes or signs of an enlarged heart on physical examination or on the electrocardiogram or chest X ray), a diagnosis of hypertension is justified and treatment should be started without waiting for a repeat reading or examination. For most patients, however, subsequent blood pressure measurements are needed to determine whether they do, indeed, have hypertension that requires specific nondrug or drug treatment.

Typically, if moderately elevated blood pressures are found, say, in the range of 140–160/90–100, and there are no signs of blood vessel damage, the patient is asked to return for follow-up measurements in about three months. There is little danger to the patient with this delayed approach. In the meantime, simple life-style modifications that may help lower the elevated levels to normal are advised. These include cutting back on salt intake, starting a modified exercise program, losing any excess weight, reducing alcohol intake if it exceeds more than three ounces a day, and limiting the intake of coffee and other sources of caffeine to the equivalent of two or three cups a day. Although the relationship between smoking and hypertension is unclear, it is well known that tobacco use greatly increases the risk of blood vessel disease and heart attacks as well as certain cancers, lung disease and other serious diseases. Thus, I strongly advise patients who smoke to make every effort to stop.

On the follow-up visit blood pressure will again be measured several times. If it is still in the less severe range (above 140/90 but under 150–155/95–100), the patient might again be advised to continue the nondrug treatments described above for another two or three months. If, at the end of this period, the blood pressure remains at levels higher than 140/190, specific blood pressure-lowering medication should be started. (Typical anti-hypertensive drug regimens are described in Chapter 7.)

This is a cautious, somewhat low-key approach, one that some patients may question in view of the potentially serious consequences of hypertension. But numerous medical studies and my own extensive experience in treating such patients support it. For the majority of hypertensive patients (about 70 percent), elevated blood pressure is in the less severe range, not to be ignored, but not a cause for overreaction either. It usually progresses slowly, and a three- or four-month delay in beginning specific treatment with medication is not dangerous to the patient. Before initiating lifelong drug therapy, I want to make sure that hypertension is indeed present and that it cannot be controlled by moderate life-style changes.

Some physicians view even *this* approach as too aggressive and don't initiate drug treatment unless blood pressure remains above 145–150/95–100 mmHg. I strongly disagree with this and will discuss later why I believe that treatment is justified when diastolic pressure levels are consistently above 90 and that delaying therapy until levels are at 95 or 100 is a mistake.

Exceptions to this low-key approach would include patients who have blood pressures above 150–160/100–110 or clear evidence of hypertension-related organ damage (i.e., an enlarged heart or evidence of kidney problems). These exceptions usually are readily apparent in the initial examination; very few patients will require extensive test procedures unless a specific cause of the hypertension is suspected. As noted, treatment begins earlier in these cases.

At-Home Measurements

During the diagnostic process patients frequently ask whether they should also have their blood pressures checked at home or at work. While this probably does no harm in most instances, it is not an important factor in the diagnostic process and, in fact, may be misleading. In recent years we have heard a good deal about so-called white-coat hypertension. This refers to the fact that people often have elevated pressures in a doctor's office yet have normal readings at home or work. There has been some debate over whether a person whose blood pressure is elevated only in a doctor's office is actually hypertensive and whether he or she should undergo any treatment at all. Why, the argument goes, treat someone if his or her blood pressure is normal most of the time? The fact is, all medical studies on high blood pressure and its consequences have been based on data collected in a physician's office, a clinic, or a medical research setting. And these indicate that a "casual" reading is a valid predictor. We have no data on the predictive accuracy of home blood pressure measurements. In other words, if repeated measurements in a doctor's office confirm that blood pressure is too high, there is probably a valid basis for treatment.

Studies many years ago involved Army recruits. During their induction physical examinations they wandered around partially dressed, being poked at by strange doctors and worried about what would happen next. They all were nervous, yet only about 15 percent of them had elevated blood pressures. Why was this so? It was because their nervous systems reacted differently from the other 85 percent of young men. Over the next ten to fifteen years a higher percentage of the 15 percent whose blood pressures became elevated under these nerve-racking circumstances developed persistently higher blood pressures than those whose pressures had remained normal during the induction ordeal. In other words, *blood pressures taken when people are anxious or worried tell us something about their futures.* So-called white-coat pressures are not to be ignored. Just one reading may be predictive, but as noted, a treatment decision should not be based on that one reading.

Twenty-four-Hour Blood Pressure Monitoring

In recent years some physicians have advocated the use of twenty-four-hour blood pressure monitors, either as part of the diagnostic process or to evaluate the effectiveness of treatment. According to the most recent guidelines from the National High Blood Pressure Education Program, ". . . for the majority of hypertensive patients, such ambulatory monitoring is not recommended for diagnosis and follow-up." I heartily concur with this view.

Not all my medical colleagues agree. Some urge patients to be hooked up to twenty-four-hour blood pressure monitors. To the unsuspecting patient, this may seem like a reasonable suggestion. After all, wouldn't it be useful to know exactly what goes on over the course of an entire day? Despite the apparent logic, there is no evidence that twenty-four-hour monitoring is any better than periodic blood pressure checks in a doctor's office or at home. It is an expensive test (two hundred to three hundred dollars) that, in the vast majority of cases, does not alter the approach to treatment. Thus, for the typical patient there is no justification for twenty-four-hour blood pressure monitors. As noted elsewhere, blood pressures do fluctuate from minute to minute and follow a pattern—lowest from midnight to 6:00 A.M., high from 6:00 A.M. to 8:00 P.M., with a gradual decrease from 8:00 P.M. to midnight, but we do not have to document this in every patient. Blood pressure monitoring is useful in research settings to determine the duration of action of a new medication, but its use at present should probably be reserved for research purposes. If a patient or a physician wants to get a handle on pressures outside an office setting, blood pressures can be taken at home or at work once every week or two for a while. But in the majority of cases treatment can be pursued effectively without this.

Exercise Tolerance Tests

Many physicians advocate that a hypertensive patient undergo an exercise tolerance, or stress, test with an electrocardiogram (ECG) prior to treatment. The rationale is that this test helps identify those patients who may have previously undetected coronary artery disease. The individual performing the test rides a bicycle or walks on a treadmill at increasing speeds until the heart rate is raised to 125 to 150 beats a minute, depending on the patient's age. If the arteries to the heart muscle are narrowed, they will not be able to dilate (or enlarge) enough to deliver the amount of blood and oxygen necessary to sustain the rapid rate and increased heart work, and a change on the ECG will be noted. The rise in blood pressure during exercise gives an indication of how labile (variable) the pressure is. Pressures normally will rise from 120–130/80 to about 160–170/85–85 at maximum exercise. Pressures that go to 200–210/95–110 or higher suggest an overreactive response, the beginning of hypertension, or poor overall control of blood pressure. In my experience, an exercise test is rarely necessary however, to aid in the diagnosis or initiation of blood pressure-lowering medication. It's simply another one of those expensive tests that doctors frequently layer onto the more necessary studies. As noted elsewhere, there are situations where this test is useful. If it is deemed important, however, to determine how exercise affects a patient's blood pressure, a doctor can, during a routine office visit, have the patient hop up and down fifty or a hundred times or jog in place for three or four minutes. This will usually provide much of the desired information without the expense (about two hundred dollars or more) or anxiety that may result from a full-scale exercise stress test.

In about 15 to 20 percent of men and an even higher percentage of women, an exercise stress test may suggest abnormalities that do not exist. This is known as a false positive test. These falsely abnormal results are common in individuals with hypertension, and unfortunately we cannot easily separate the false positives from true positives without more tests. Such tests may include a thallium (radionuclide) stress test or coronary angiography. The latter is a complicated, costly examination in which a catheter is threaded through a blood vessel in either the groin or the arm and into the heart itself. A dye is injected into the circulation to make the coronary arteries show up on X-ray film. This examination costs about twelve hundred to fifteen hundred dollars, and more important, it carries a small but definite risk of producing vascular complications. It can also be emotionally truumatic for the patient. Such an examination should not be entered into lightly. It is an extremely useful test, but there should be a clear indication that it is needed *and* that the information gained from it will be helpful in the design of a treatment program.

When, then, is an exercise stress test justified? I recommend it for patients who have symptoms, such as chest pains or shortness of breath that do not fit into a classic pattern of angina pectoris (or "typical" chest pains from heart disease). It also may be justified for sedentary people who wish to begin *vigorous* conditioning programs, especially if they have cardiovascular risk factors, such as tobacco use, high blood pressure, high blood cholesterol, and so forth. I do *not* consider it necessary for patients who have been exercising all along without symptoms, and I certainly do not advise it as part of an initial examination of patients with high blood pressure or, indeed, as part of a routine physical examination in people without symptoms.

Echocardiograms

The echocardiogram is yet another overused diagnostic study that has only limited usefulness for hypertensive patients. This examination uses sound waves to map internal organs. It is noninvasive, does not hurt, has no complications, and takes about thirty to sixty minutes to perform. There is no question that it can detect an enlarged heart—a complication of long-standing high blood pressure—at an earlier stage than an electrocardiogram. The fact remains, however, that for the typical hypertensive patient the findings on an echocardiogram will not change the approach to therapy. I rarely advise use of this test in the initial study of a person with hypertension. If blood pressures are above 150–160/100, for example, medications are indicated *even* if the electrocardiogram and physical examination fail to show evidence of heart enlargement. If blood pressures are between 140–150/90–100, some physicians delay specific treatment unless there is evidence of heart enlargement. I do not agree with this. These patients should be treated whether or not the heart is enlarged. Data from a major study, the Hypertension Detection and Follow-Up Program Study, show that if you wait until evidence of heart enlargement is present, treatment is not nearly as successful in reducing risk of a stroke or heart attack as it is when treatment is begun earlier. It may be of academic interest to a physician to have the *exact* information obtained from an echocardiogram, but it isn't usually necessary, and the cost, which ranges from two hundred to three hundred fifty dollars, may be more than enough to pay for a typical year's therapy. A good general rule to follow is that if a test result is not going to change an approach to treatment significantly, then it just may not be necessary, especially if the procedure is expensive, anxiety-provoking, or painful.

Before agreeing to any major medical test, like a stress test or echocardiogram, the patient should ask why the procedure is needed and how the information will alter treatment. If this question cannot be answered satisfactorily, there is probably no good reason to do the test. Answers like "We're doing it to be complete" and

"To get an idea of what your heart really looks like" are not sufficient justification for the test. Perhaps someday, if an echocardiogram can be performed at lower cost, its wider use in patients with high blood pressure can be advocated.

Special Circumstances

More than 90 percent of all cases of hypertension have no clinically identifiable cause. This type of high blood pressure is known as primary, or essential, hypertension, and the diagnostic process described above is adequate for most of these patients. There are, however, unusual instances in which high blood pressure may be secondary to a specific disorder, and in these cases additional tests are needed to identify the cause. It should be stressed that although we cannot cure primary hypertension, we can treat it and prevent problems. In the following instances, however, we may be able to find a specific cause for elevated blood pressure, remove it, and cure the disease.

ADRENAL TUMORS

The two adrenal glands, which are situated on top of the kidneys, produce a number of hormones. One of these is called aldosterone, a steroid hormone that helps control the body's chemical balance by helping the kidneys conserve sodium. This hormone also regulates the excretion of potassium, another essential mineral of the body. If the adrenal glands secrete excessive amounts of aldosterone, the body retains too much sodium and loses too much potassium. This leads to an increase in the amount of fluid in tissues and blood vessels, which then causes the heart to work harder and the blood vessels to contract. As a result, blood pressure is increased. The excessive aldosterone is due either to a small adrenal tumor or to a general overactivity of the adrenal glands. This type of hypertension may be accompanied by various symptoms—specifically, muscle weakness or excessive urination or thirst. A blood test may show low potassium levels. If your doctor suspects this as the cause of your hypertension, he or she may do hormone studies on the blood or urine or a CAT scan, which is a computerized X-ray study that outlines body organs and can detect even small tumors of the adrenal glands. You also may be hospitalized for a day or two and given several intravenous tests.

If a specific tumor is diagnosed, it can be removed and the hypertension is usually cured. The tumors are rarely malignant. If overactive adrenal glands without a tumor are present, the treatment is medicinal—specific drugs are used to block the activity of aldosterone—and pressure can be controlled as long as medication is used. Remember, this form of hypertension is extremely rare (less than one half of 1 percent of all hypertensives), and it is usually not necessary to do studies to find it.

HYPERTENSION CAUSED BY KIDNEY PROBLEMS

Since the kidneys are so important in regulating blood pressure, it follows that any chronic kidney disorder may cause hypertension. Special kidney studies may be indicated in cases of high blood pressure that do not respond to standard treatment and in patients with certain symptoms or physical findings. Kidney disorders also should be suspected in very young patients with hypertension and in patients with diabetes.

Disorders of the kidney represent about 4 percent

of all cases of hypertension, making it the most common form of secondary hypertension (hypertension with a specific cause). There are several reasons for this. People with chronic kidney disorders (for example, long-standing, recurrent infections) may have compromised kidney function that leads to hypertension. This is occasionally seen in women who have had repeated urinary tract or bladder infections. After many infections the kidneys may fail to function adequately and blood pressure may gradually rise.

In some instances hypertension may be noted many years after an episode of nephritis, a kidney infection caused by streptococcal bacteria. Fortunately nephritis is much less common today than in the past, thanks to the use of antibiotics to control infections in young children.

Diabetes can cause progressive narrowing of the blood vessels in the kidneys and other tissue changes that eventually reduce the kidney's ability to excrete salt and water effectively, thus leading to fluid retention that raises blood pressure.

Simple urine tests can rule out many cases of kidney-related hypertension. For example, urine normally contains very little protein because a filter in the kidneys prevents protein from leaking out of the blood into the urine. In a damaged kidney, however, some of the protein leaks past a defective filtering system and shows up in the urine. High levels of protein in the urine may indicate either a chronic infection or progressive kidney disease. In addition, a microscopic examination of the urine will often reveal the presence of red or white blood cells—another sign of a kidney infection or chronic kidney disease.

In the case of diabetes, hypertension usually is not an early finding; your physician should be able to diagnose kidney disease secondary to diabetes on the basis of a medical history, urine and blood tests, and the presence of high blood pressure.

At one time hypertension related to kidney disease was considered a fatal form of the disease. Today many patients, even including those with long-standing kidney disease and evidence of decreased kidney function, can be treated satisfactorily. Several of the blood pressure-lowering drugs are effective in these cases. I have followed many patients with kidney disease *caused* by neglected hypertension, as well as others who had kidney disease *resulting* in hypertension. Once their blood pressures were lowered, they did well for many years. Unfortunately about 25 percent of patients who end up in dialysis programs in the United States started out with "mild" hypertension that progressed because blood pressure was not lowered. A similar circumstance prevails in diabetic patients whose disease is poorly controlled. They *may* end up on dialysis, but they stand a much better chance of delaying this if their blood pressures are controlled—in fact this may be more important in preventing kidney disease than control of blood sugar.

RENOVASCULAR HYPERTENSION

An interesting form of hypertension secondary to kidney disease is renovascular disease, or high blood pressure caused by a narrowed renal (kidney) artery. The aorta branches just about at the level of the mid-abdomen or navel into the renal or kidney arteries—one for each kidney. If a narrowing occurs in one or both of these renal arteries, less blood is supplied to kidney tissue and the affected kidney secretes excessive amounts of the hormone called renin. Narrowing is usually caused by a fatty plaque in older persons and by a type of inflammation in younger ones. Renin, through a series of

reactions and enzyme changes, produces a powerful substance called angiotensin II, which can cause marked
constriction of blood vessels as well as increased excretion of aldosterone, the adrenal hormone discussed
above. As a result, the patient ends up with excessive
retention of salt and water and with hypertension.

This condition should be suspected in any young
person (under the age of fifteen years) who develops
hypertension, and appropriate diagnostic studies should
be carried out. Renovascular hypertension also should
be suspected in an older person whose high blood pressure has been controlled for many years and then gets
out of control for no apparent reason. It also is a possibility in people over sixty who have had documented
normal blood pressures most of their lives and who then
develop hypertension. One way of detecting renovascular hypertension is by special X-ray studies in which a dye
is injected into a vein to help visualize the kidneys. The
X rays will show whether the kidneys are getting enough
blood. A more definitive study involves the insertion of
a catheter into an artery in the groin and the injection of
dye directly into the renal arteries. Narrowing, if found,
can be corrected either by insertion of a catheter with a
balloon and expansion of the balloon to widen the vessel
or by a surgical procedure in which the blocked blood
vessel is bypassed by an artificial graft.

An unusual type of renovascular disease is found in
young women (and occasionally in men) in whom the
artery narrowing is caused by an inflammatory change in
the muscles encircling the blood vessel. These muscles
harden in rings and make the artery look like a bamboo
shoot. This can be treated by insertion of a balloon catheter and expansion of the artery enough to crack the
little bands of hardened muscle and open up the artery.
Seven years ago I saw a thirteen-year-old girl with this

type of inflammatory renovascular hypertension. Her blood pressure was 180/100; but her serum potassium level was normal, ruling out the possibility of a tumor of the adrenal gland, and she had no symptoms to suggest an excessive amount of adrenaline. I did an arteriographic examination, injecting dye and visualizing her kidney arteries. She showed a narrowing of both renal arteries typical of this type of inflammatory disorder. Over the course of the next two weeks, both arteries were opened up by a balloon catheter (angioplasty), and her blood pressure became normal. After six years her blood pressure is still normal, and she requires no medication. If I had not looked for and found this lesion, the young woman would have had to remain on medication the rest of her life. I might have been able to control her blood pressure, but it certainly was easier this way.

There is no guarantee that blood pressure will return to normal in every case, but the success rate is 70 to 80 percent in the muscular inflammatory type and about 40 to 50 percent in other patients with renovascular hypertension.

PHEOCHROMOCYTOMA

This is a rare condition in which a tumor produces excessive amounts of epinephrine and norepinephrine, hormones which are normally secreted by the adrenal glands. These hormones, commonly referred to as adrenaline, are important in the body's fight-or-flight response; they speed up the heartbeat and raise blood pressure. Patients with pheochromocytoma usually have at least one or more specific symptoms related to the excessive amounts of adrenaline; palpitations, headaches, tremors, feelings of agitation, pallor, cold, clammy skin, and inappropriate sweating of the face, back, or chest in a cool room. They may faint upon standing up. Symptoms and/or high blood pressure may not be present all the time. In fact, some patients have normal blood pressure more often than not. About 90 percent of these funny-sounding tumors develop on the adrenal glands, but they can also be found in other parts of the body, along the aorta, near the spine or in the chest, or in the bladder.

One of the first medical articles I wrote described a patient with pheochromocytoma, a forty-two-year-old black man who had been hospitalized for a gallbladder operation. The chart said he had normal blood pressure, but when I checked him on his preoperative examination, I found that his blood pressure was an astounding 250/140. His face was covered with sweat, his pulse was rapid; his skin felt cold and clammy. He said he had spells like this several times a day but felt normal in between. In my then-short career I had never encountered anything like this, so I immediately headed for the medical library. I ran across a description of pheochromocytoma and decided that this must be what was bothering the patient.

I alerted the patient's surgeon, who was reluctant to cancel the operation. A nurse had also taken the patient's blood pressure about an hour after I had, and it was normal; but a few hours later it was rechecked, and sure enough, it was again in the 250/140 range. The diagnosis of pheochromocytoma was confirmed by several tests, and removal of the hormone-producing tumor cured the episodes of high blood pressure. The patient's so-called gallstones turned out to be deposits of calcium in the tumor.

Sometimes these tumors are detected accidentally. Examining the abdomen and pressing the side where a pheochromocytoma is located may cause an outpouring of adrenaline and a marked rise in blood pressure and pulse rate. Generally these are small tumors, but they can be detected by a CAT scan or other X-ray studies. A simple screening test will be ordered if a pheo-chromocytoma is suspected on the basis of the medical history or physical exam. A twenty-four-hour urine collection will be suggested to determine the amount of adrenaline. If this shows increased amounts, further studies will be done.

Surgical removal of the tumor will usually cure high blood pressure unless it has been present for many years. These tumors are occasionally malignant (about 10 percent). Drugs such as the alpha blockers like prazosin (Minipress) or phenoxybenzamine (Dibenzyline), with or without a beta blocker, that inhibit the sympathetic nervous system (the system that controls heart rate and constriction of blood vessels) may be given to lower the blood pressure pending surgical treatment. Remember, this tumor is also extremely rare (less than one half of one percent of all cases), and routine studies to search for it are not necessary.

COARCTATION OF THE AORTA

This is a rather rare congenital defect in which part of the aorta is narrowed after it leaves the heart and after it branches off into the major arteries of the neck and arm. It is seen more commonly in males and usually is apparent in early childhood (if it is looked for), though in some instances it may not be detected until the second or third decades of life. Blood pressures may not be very high—i.e., 140–150/90–95. Pulses in the arms are good, but because the narrowing results in less blood flow to the legs, the pulses in the groin or leg arteries are faint or even absent. A diagnosis of coarctation should be made on physical examination and confirmed by X-ray studies. The narrowing can be repaired surgically with good results.

CUSHING'S DISEASE

There is another extremely rare cause of hypertension that is related to an excess of adrenal or steroid hormones. Patients with Cushing's disease are usually obese, usually have diabetes and a hump of tissue on the upper back just below the neck (commonly referred to as a buffalo hump), and have other distinguishing characteristics. Hormone studies will confirm this diagnosis.

MISCELLANEOUS

Other causes of secondary hypertension include the use of certain drugs, such as birth control pills, prolonged use of steroid hormones like cortisone (prednisone) and certain other prescription drugs such as medications used for arthritis as well as some nonprescription cold remedies, appetite suppressants, and nasal decongestants. You should always tell your doctor about any medications, both prescription and over-the-counter, that you are taking. It is not often that they actually cause hypertension, but they may aggravate it in patients with "mild hypertension" or may interfere somewhat with the actions of some of the blood pressure-lowering drugs.

Finally, there are a few rare cases of high blood pressure that can be traced to a simple, easily eliminated cause; finding the cause may require some detective work. I recall the case of a forty-two-year-old secretary who had recently developed quite high blood pressures (155–165/105–110). She was not taking birth control pills, and she was in excellent general health. She religiously cut back on salt, but her pressures stayed up. On her second office visit I detected a smell of licorice on her breath. Questioning revealed that yes, she was very fond of licorice. In fact, she had recently gotten a package of several pounds of licorice from her relations in Finland and had been nibbling on licorice sticks quite a lot over the past month.

Licorice contains glycyrrhizic acid, a compound that promotes sodium retention and acts like one of the adrenal hormones. Large amounts of glycyrrhizic acid can raise blood pressure. Since most licorice candy in the United States is now made with artificial flavoring, we don't see much high blood pressure related to it these days. But the Europeans still use the real thing, and that's what my patient was eating. I suspected licorice was causing her high blood pressure and urged her to stop eating it. In less than a week her blood pressure was back to normal.

There may be other unusual causes of high blood pressure, but they are even rarer than the ones we have cited. Remember, most everyone has the kind of hypertension that may not be *curable* but can be treated successfully with good results.

Summing Up

• A diagnosis of hypertension usually requires several blood pressure readings. Factors such as stress, caffeine, or nicotine can produce a misleadingly high reading. Higher pressures when someone is nervous are, however, usually valid as predictors of future high blood pressure.

• Twenty-four-hour blood pressure monitoring, stress tests, and echocardiograms are usually not necessary for the proper evaluation of a patient with hypertension.

• Hospitalization is rarely necessary for a person with high blood pressure.

• The relatively rare cases of secondary hypertension can usually be found if certain guidelines are followed.

• Acceptable treatment for hypertension means *controlling* blood pressure levels, not simply taking medication, which may not be effective.

3

THE EFFECTS OF HIGH BLOOD PRESSURE

Earlier we reviewed the tragic consequences of President Roosevelt's uncontrolled high blood pressure. While this is an extreme case, one that we would be unlikely to see today, it does illustrate the kind of damage that hypertension can cause to a number of organ systems. In this chapter the effects of high blood pressure on these target organs will be described. I will also outline a commonsense preventive approach which can protect the tissues most susceptible to the effects of high blood pressure.

The Blood Vessels

Arteries are composed of several layers of different tissues. The inner layer is composed of endothelial cells. Normally these cells form a smooth surface, similar to the lining of the mouth, and they are sealed together so that only the smallest microscopic particles can seep beneath the surface lining. The outer layer of the artery serves as a wrapper, and the middle layer, which consists of muscle, gives the artery its elasticity—the ability to dilate or contract. The blood vessels that are affected by elevated blood pressure include both the larger arteries—like the aorta and its branches, which carry blood to the arms, legs, kidneys, and other organs—and the smaller vessels within the kidney, heart, and brain. In other words, hypertension affects almost all arteries of the body but in different ways.

The exact process by which hypertension damages the large blood vessels and speeds up the process of hardening of the arteries is not fully understood, but some researchers believe that the long-standing high pressure of blood moving through these vessels damages the artery walls and the cells that form their surface linings. Certain components of the blood, especially fatty substances like cholesterol—which we all have in various amounts within the blood system—can then seep through these tiny cracks in the endothelial lining, forming clumps of fatty material (or plaque) beneath the surface. This is comparable to the rust that accumulates inside plumbing pipes. The more cholesterol in the bloodstream, the more "rust" forms in the damaged vessels.

Not everyone believes that high blood pressure specifically injures the material that binds these lining cells together. Some scientists have found evidence to suggest that elevated blood pressure produces a type of inflammatory reaction beneath the artery wall surface and that this inflammation is what damages the endothelial lining. In any event, the vessel becomes roughened and narrowed. This represents the process of atherosclerosis, the medical term for a type of hardening of the arteries characterized by deposits of fatty material. As fatty deposits build up, the vessel narrows, and less and less blood is able to flow through it to the tissues it supplies. In the case of the brain or heart, even a small decrease in the blood supply may produce some symptoms.

Platelets, a component of the blood important to clot formation, accumulate in the damaged areas of a blood vessel. The clumping or sticking together of platelets results in the formation of a clot (or thrombus) which can completely block an artery. Clot formation is obviously an important way to stop bleeding when we cut ourselves, and this is an important function of the platelets. If we didn't have platelets, as well as other clot-promoting substances, we could bleed to death from a simple cut. *But* if a clot forms in an artery which supplies blood to the heart (a coronary artery), a heart attack is the likely result. A stroke can be caused by a clot in an artery that supplies the brain (a cerebral blood vessel). Depending upon where the clot forms, the stroke may be temporary and small, with only minimal weakness or other symptoms; in other instances it may be full blown, with lasting effects that can include paralysis or even death.

Chronic high blood pressure also affects the layer of muscle that encircles the arteries. (See Figure 1.) Studies in animals with hypertension have found that the arterioles—the smaller arteries which have a lot of muscle tissue and which can contract or expand easily—have a thicker than normal layer of muscle. In the tissues of humans with long-standing hypertension, the smaller arteries also become thickened and narrowed. When this happens in the kidney, kidney function may decrease significantly which results in a backing up of waste products.

Long-standing hypertension may also result in the weakening or thinning of the walls of the arteries. When this happens in the larger arteries, such as the aorta, an aneurysm—a blisterlike weakened segment of the artery—may result. This resembles a balloonlike expansion of a weakened inner tube of a tire. To envision how this happens, let's go back to the analogy of the garden hose and faucet. If you turn the faucet on and off, you intermittently raise and lower the pressure in the hose.

When the nozzle is left open, every time you fully open the faucet there is some increase in water pressure in the hose, but not as much as if the nozzle is closed. When the nozzle remains closed and you keep the faucet open, the increasing water pressure may cause a ballooning out *if a portion of the rubber hose is rotted or defective.* Eventually a tear or rip may develop in this area. Similarly, an aneurysm may occur in a weakened or damaged area of a blood vessel if blood pressure is too high, the vessel may then rupture. Fortunately our blood vessels are quite strong, and it takes a lot of wear and tear to thin them out or weaken them; they can withstand increased pressure for many years. But if high blood pressure is left untreated and an aneurysm happens to form in a blood vessel in the brain, for example, a rupture can cause a stroke or even death. Such a rupture is called a cerebral hemorrhage. A rupture of the aorta—the great artery that arises from the heart and branches out to carry blood to the upper and lower parts of the body—can result in fatal hemorrhaging. Occasionally the tear in the vessel only affects its inner lining, and the blood can dissect through the middle of the artery without causing a full rupture.

If the arteries in the legs become narrowed or clogged with fatty material, blood flow to the legs decreases, and a condition called intermittent claudication may result. This may appear in older people with long-standing high blood pressure and other risk factors who have developed arteriosclerosis or in individuals with long-standing diabetes. Claudication is characterized by pains in the calves or thighs which occur while walking or climbing stairs. These pains subside after a few minutes of rest, and activity can then be resumed. They are similar to the chest pains experienced by persons with narrowed arteries to the heart, a condition called angina

FIGURE 1: *How Untreated High Blood Pressure Can Harm Various Organ Systems*

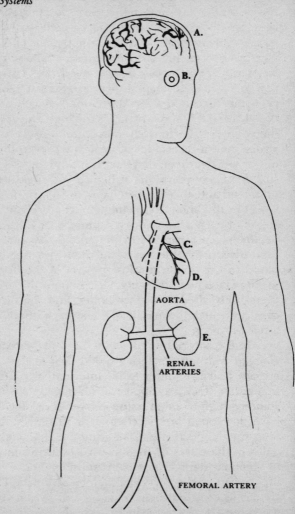

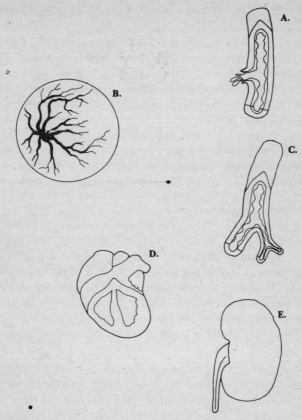

A. The brain: High blood pressure may weaken blood vessels, resulting in hemorrhage and a stroke, or it may hasten hardening of the arteries, which may result in
a clot and a stroke

B. The eye: Tiny arteries may become thickened and narrowed, leading to vision loss

C. Coronary arteries: May become narrowed and clogged with fatty deposits, leading
to angina and increasing the risk of a heart attack.

D. The heart: Muscle walls may become thickened, reducing the heart's ability to
pump blood and increasing the risk of heart failure

E. The kidney: Blood vessels may become narrowed, reducing the kidney's ability to
filter out waste products from the blood

pectoris (pain in the chest). People with intermittent claudication or angina usually learn by experience how far they can walk without difficulty, and in fact, walking up to tolerance is good for them. It helps open up new, little collateral blood vessels that carry blood around the area of narrowing or blockage. In effect, a person who develops good collateral circulation does his or her own nonsurgical bypass.

While hypertension is not the major factor responsible for angina or poor circulation in the legs, it is an important risk factor for early arteriosclerosis (hardening of the arteries) which contributes to these conditions.

The Heart

As you might imagine, the heart itself is one of the major organs affected by uncontrolled high blood pressure. People with hypertension have a higher incidence of heart attacks than those without, although heart attacks also occur in people with normal blood pressure. There are two basic ways in which high blood pressure affects the heart.

1. As noted, hypertension speeds up the process of atherosclerosis. This may result in a narrowing of the arteries that supply blood to the heart muscle, the coronary arteries.

2. Chronic high blood pressure can lead to an enlarged heart. The increased pressure causes the heart to work harder—it must beat more forcefully than normal—and since the heart itself is made up mostly of muscle tissue (the myocardium), increased work will enlarge it. We all know that if we exercise our muscles regularly, they become larger, a phenomenon amply demonstrated by the effects of weight lifting. A similar phenomenon takes place in a heart that is chronically overworked.

In a person with high blood pressure the heart is forced to work harder simply to get enough blood to such vital organs as the brain and kidney, and so the heart muscle becomes thicker. Initially this is not harmful. It is the heart's way of ensuring that it meets the increased demands placed on it by chronically increased blood pressure. If high blood pressure remains untreated, however, the enlarged heart eventually becomes less efficient. There may be too little blood passing through its own arteries to nourish the extra amount of muscle.

The enlarged hearts of the chronically hypertensive differ from the enlarged hearts frequently seen in marathon runners. These athletes' hearts often develop extra collateral blood vessels in order to nourish the increased mass of muscle, and they also become superefficient at extracting oxygen from the blood. The enlarged hearts of the chronically hypertensive, however, often lack an adequate blood supply. For one thing, hypertensive individuals tend to be middle-aged or older, and their coronary arteries are more likely to be narrowed by atherosclerosis. This diminishes their ability to nourish the overworked and thickened heart muscle. In addition, the hearts of those over sixty tend to be less resilient and are therefore less efficient at pumping blood.

The part of the heart that is most affected by chronic hypertension is the left ventricle, the main pumping chamber. The entire heart may be enlarged, but it is the enlargement of the left ventricle (a condition called left ventricular hypertrophy) that is particularly serious. If the left ventricle becomes too thick, it may fail to pump out enough blood with each beat, excess blood may back up into the lungs, the lungs become water-logged, and shortness of breath results. This is called congestive heart failure. In addition, body tissues may become waterlogged (a condition known as edema), causing the feet and legs to swell.

An enlarged heart is also more susceptible to ir-regular beats (arrhythmias). Again, lack of blood supply to certain areas of the heart may cause an irritability and "extra beats," which are often perceived by patients as missed or skipped beats or palpitations.

It generally takes many years for an enlarged heart caused by hypertension to progress to a serious stage. Early diagnosis and treatment of high blood pressure can prevent heart enlargement and heart failure as well as other serious consequences of hypertension. Heart failure caused by hypertension used to be a commonly noted illness. Today it is rare. In my practice it has been more than fifteen years since I have seen a case of heart failure in a person with hypertension, mainly because the condition is treated early and the pressure is kept as close to normal as possible. There is also good evidence that treating high blood pressure can actually reverse heart enlargement and return the heart to normal size.

Unfortunately, some popular publications persist in saying, "a little hypertension is not harmful and may even be beneficial." This opinion is based upon the mis-taken belief that in some persons, whose arteries to the brain and kidney may be narrowed, a greater head of pressure is necessary to force blood into these organs. This theory is false and potentially dangerous to people who believe and act on it, for by doing so, they may end up with not only more than just a little high blood pres-sure but evidence of "target organ" (heart, kidney, or brain) damage as well. Persistent high blood pressure damages and narrows blood vessels.

I recall one patient who came to my office about six years ago. At the time he was forty-seven years old, and his blood pressure was 145/95—not very high, but in a range that should have been treated. This patient, J. T., had read some articles which suggested that mild degrees of high blood pressure need not be bothered with, as long as the person felt good, and that some of the blood pressure-lowering drugs might actually be harmful. He was determined to try "natural" methods to lower his blood pressure and to stay away from "toxic" drugs, especially since he was convinced by his reading that a little high blood pressure wasn't so bad. He embarked on an exercise program, restricted his salt intake, stopped smoking, and cut down on his usual alcohol intake of three or four drinks a day. In other words, he did all the things that most physicians recommend as initial therapy.

All these are reasonable approaches to treatment, and in some people they are adequate to lower the less severe levels of high blood pressure to normal, at least for a period of time. Unfortunately J. T. did not fall into this lucky category. When he returned to the office five years later, he had not seen a physician in the intervening time, and his blood pressure had risen to 155/105—still not a dangerous level but obviously higher than before. There also was evidence of organ damage. His electrocardiogram and chest X ray showed that now his heart was enlarged. Urine tests showed some protein, an early sign of kidney damage. These tests had been normal five years before. Fortunately, this time, we were able to convince him to go on specific medication to lower his blood pressure. We started with a diuretic, which was sufficient to bring his pressure down to normal. After six months on this therapy we compared his ECG and chest X ray to the earlier ones and found that his heart size actually was returning to normal. The protein in the urine had disappeared.

I don't know exactly how many patients I have seen over the past 35 years whose heart sizes have returned to normal after proper treatment of their blood pressures, but in my last review of more than five hundred cases in 1987, almost 50 percent of those with hypertensive heart disease and an enlarged heart had experienced a decrease in heart size as blood pressure was lowered and maintained at normal or near-normal levels. All the drugs that are currently recommended as possible *initial* therapy have been shown to be effective in reducing heart size—if blood pressure is reduced. The message is clear: Treat before evidence of heart or kidney damage, *but* even if treatment is delayed for one reason or another, some of the damage can be repaired.

The Kidneys

The kidneys are among the hardest-working organs in the body. They have a network of tiny filtering structures called nephrons. Blood constantly flows through these nephrons, where the waste products of body metabolism are filtered out and excreted in the urine. If the tiny blood vessels in the kidneys become narrowed and damaged by high blood pressure, blood flow to the nephrons is reduced and the kidneys are unable to eliminate waste products efficiently. These may back up in the blood and can be detected by simple blood tests for blood urea nitrogen (BUN) and creatinine—both byproducts of protein metabolism. Fortunately, as with the heart, the kidneys are quite resistant to injury, and it may take years for blood vessel changes to affect kidney function adversely. This may occur more quickly in a person with hypertension and diabetes and is seen more commonly in the elderly.

If the nephrons are severely damaged by chronic high blood pressure (or other conditions such as diabetes or recurrent infections), waste products build up in the blood and may result in a condition called uremia (kidney failure). It is important to note that people can go on for many years with lesser degrees of kidney failure. Eventually in some of them, if symptoms of weakness and anemia develop, kidney dialysis may become necessary. This is an expensive, time-consuming, and uncomfortable treatment in which the patient is attached to a machine for several hours, two to four times a week, in order to filter the blood mechanically. Still, we're fortunate to have this kind of treatment available, for thousands of people have had their lives prolonged or saved by dialysis. We should remember that one out of every four or five dialysis patients had, at one point, just "mild" high blood pressure, but that as a result of poor or inadequate treatment, the elevated blood pressure led to kidney failure. This has been especially true in the black population. *Early control of high blood pressure usually can prevent this type of kidney failure.* Many millions of dollars plus all the discomfort to this portion of the dialysis population, could be saved yearly if only hypertension were treated more effectively at an early stage in more people.

Considering the high cost of kidney dialysis and the less than satisfactory quality of life endured by most dialysis patients, prevention is obviously vastly preferable to letting high blood pressure progress to kidney failure. Unfortunately the press continues to publish articles that "warn" of the dangers of blood pressure-lowering drugs and their possible adverse effects on the kidney. One of our most effective antihypertensive medications, the diuretic, has been labeled as just such a medication. Nothing could be further from the truth. Numerous well-controlled scientific studies have shown exactly the opposite, that hypertensive patients treated with diuretics (and other blood pressure-lowering medications) have a *reduced* incidence of kidney failure. In my experience even patients with early evidence of kidney damage improve when their blood pressures are brought under control.

I am always upset when I'm asked to see patients who have been poorly treated because of the fear that medication might hurt their weakened kidneys. To be sure, caution must be used in lowering blood pressure when there is already evidence of kidney damage, and some medications may be contraindicated. But in general, getting blood pressure down to normal *prevents,* rather than speeds up, further reduction in kidney function. I have seen numerous patients with advanced kidney disease manage well for many years once their blood pressures were controlled. In some, dialysis does become necessary, but its use was probably delayed for years by blood pressure treatment. Recent evidence also strongly suggests that in diabetic patients who have hypertension and kidney problems, the lowering of blood pressure slows down the progression of kidney damage and may even improve function.

The Brain

A steady supply of blood to the brain is vital to sustain life, and the entire circulatory system is designed to ensure this. The instant our internal communication system senses that the brain may not be getting enough blood, pressure rises and blood is diverted from other organs and sent to the brain.

Unfortunately the blood vessels that supply blood to the brain are subject to the same kind of damage from chronic high blood pressure that is seen in other parts of the body. Over time the vessels may become thicker or narrowed, and a clot may form and stop the blood flow to a specific area of the brain. This can result in a stroke, a type of stroke called, specifically, a cerebral thrombosis (brain clot). In addition, small, blisterlike aneurysms may form in one or more arteries in the brain. A rupture of one of these aneurysms can cause a hemorrhage, and this, too, can result in a type of stroke called a cerebral hemorrhage. A cerebral hemorrhage is usually more serious than a cerebral thrombosis. The carotid arteries— the major blood vessels that travel along the sides of the neck, behind the jaw, and to the brain—also can become clogged by atherosclerosis. A stroke can result if a clot blocks one of these vessels or if a piece of the clot or fatty plaque breaks away and lodges in a vessel within the brain itself (a cerebral embolus).

A stroke can be a major catastrophe. Of the estimated 500,000 Americans who suffer strokes each year, about 25 to 30 percent or 155,000 die, making it the third most common cause of death in the United States. Many of the survivors are left with varying degrees of disability, even after extensive rehabilitation. *The good news is that many strokes can be prevented.* About 70 to 80 percent of people who suffer strokes have hypertension. Since the National High Blood Pressure Education Program got under way in 1972, the number of effectively treated hypertensive patients has increased significantly, and in this same period, as noted earlier, the stroke death rate has declined by more than 50 percent. This incredible achievement has resulted in about 70,000 fewer deaths each year, *and it is due mainly to better treatment of high blood pressure.* Changes in behavioral patterns (reduction in overall use of tobacco, decreased consumption of saturated fats, and increased exercise) may also account for some of this improvement as may the use of low-dose aspirin in people at high risk for a stroke.

Frequently stroke victims experience warnings prior to a stroke in the form of ministrokes or transient ischemic attacks (TIAs). These may be due to spasms of blood vessels in the brain or to small clots. A person who has had a TIA is more likely to have a stroke at a later date than someone who has not. The symptoms of a TIA may be similar to those of a stroke: sudden weakness, clumsiness or loss of feeling in an arm, a leg, or the side of the face, loss of vision, double vision, or inability to speak. Unlike a stroke, a TIA has symptoms that last for just a few minutes or an hour or two and produce no immediately apparent damage.

Medical attention often can prevent a subsequent stroke, so it is important for anyone who has had a TIA to see a doctor. Take the case of G. S. He had had so-called mild high blood pressure for fifteen years but had not been particularly diligent about keeping it under control (not completely his fault; his doctor was one of those who were convinced that treatment was not necessary). Five years earlier, at the age of fifty-three, he had suffered a mild heart attack. As sometimes happens after a heart attack, his blood pressure returned to normal levels, but after a few years it began to creep up again, to levels of 145/95 to 150/100—not too bad but certainly too high. His first TIA occurred when he was walking to his office; he suddenly experienced severe numbness in his right leg. It passed in a few minutes, and

he put the incident out of his mind. The next day, however, he temporarily lost vision in one eye for three or
four minutes. This prompted him to call his doctor, who
told him to get to the hospital right away. Examination
showed that his blood pressure was not terribly high, at
150/90, but the doctor could hear a distinct whooshing
sound (a bruit) in one of his carotid arteries. He was
immediately put on a blood-thinning medication. Further studies showed severe narrowing in a three-inch
section of his left carotid artery. He underwent surgery
to clean out the artery (a controversial operation that
often is done without clear justification, but in this case,
symptoms warranted the procedure).

That was three years ago. G. S.'s blood pressure is
now well controlled with a diuretic and beta blocker. He
also takes one baby aspirin daily. There have been no
further symptoms, and he considers himself lucky as he
carries on an active life as a university professor.

No one can say for sure that this patient's heart
attack or ministroke would have been postponed or prevented by early and continuing treatment of his slightly
elevated blood pressure, but there is reason to believe
that it would have been less likely to occur. *In the case of
a stroke and heart attack, prevention is always easier than treatment, which is often expensive, anxiety-producing, and occasionally painful.*

Although a stroke is the most abrupt and devastating brain problem related to high blood pressure, other
disorders can take place over time. Chronic reduced
blood flow to the brain as a result of progressive narrowing of blood vessels can lead to a type of dementia. Often
the dementia is caused by multiple little strokes that
result from clots in small blood vessels; hence it is called
multi-infarct dementia. Sometimes the strokes are so
mild that they go unnoticed at the time. In such cases the

dementia may be mistaken for Alzheimer's disease, but there are important differences. Alzheimer's comes on gradually, whereas dementia related to reduced cerebral blood flow to several areas of the brain may be more rapid in its onset. Unlike Alzheimer's disease, which has no treatment, multi-infarct dementia may improve or at least remain nonprogressive if further clots are prevented. Recent studies suggest that the use of daily low-dose aspirin (a baby aspirin or one half of a regular aspirin) given early in the course of mental deterioration in certain patients may produce improvement or delay progression of symptoms. Aspirin in small doses is effective in preventing clotting. This may represent yet another use for this "old new miracle drug." Aspirin should not be used for long periods of time unless blood pressure is relatively normal.

Detecting the Effects of High Blood Pressure

Since it is possible to have high blood pressure for many years without experiencing any symptoms, it is important to be alert for signs of target-organ damage while the damage is still treatable or even reversible. So even when high blood pressure is initially diagnosed, a doctor should look for signs of possible organ damage. This usually can be accomplished with simple in-office observations; only in unusual circumstances are elaborate and expensive tests such as echocardiography, Doppler studies, kidney or blood vessel X rays, or twenty-four-hour blood pressure monitoring justified.

Unfortunately in this era of high-tech, malpractice suit-prone medicine, there is an increasing likelihood that a patient will be subjected to a battery of unnecessary tests. What's more, our insurance system (including

Medicare) plays into the hands of physicians trained to test first and think later. For example, an experienced physician would probably do more good by spending even a short time instructing a patient in effective self-care or the appropriate use of medications than by ordering a few extra reimbursible tests "just to be sure." Studies have found that patients who have had the benefit of even a few minutes of physician instruction are more likely to stop smoking, change faulty eating habits, and take medication as instructed than are patients who have not had this kind of personal counseling. Unfortunately this type of approach is not taken as often as it should be, and educational materials about high blood pressure, diabetes, and other common chronic illnesses have not been made as available as *they* should be despite recent emphasis on the "informed patient."

The fee for an office visit and a "chat" about your disease may be thirty to fifty dollars, depending upon where you live. Contrast this with the hundreds of dollars a doctor can earn in the same amount of time by doing an exercise stress test, echocardiogram, or other high-tech procedure. The present reimbursement system *rewards* physicians for procedures, *not* for their time, advice, and judgment. This should be changed. The present malpractice climate also encourages the use of procedures to protect physicians from the claims of not doing everything possible. This must also be changed.

Granted, there are instances in which these tests provide useful information that can be used to design a more effective approach to treatment, but in the management of hypertension this appears to be the exception, not the rule. And if the tests turn out to be a substitute for taking the time to talk to a patient and make simple diagnostic observations, the patient loses much more than money. He or she misses the opportunity to benefit from what should be the doctor's real mission—namely, helping the patient help himself or herself.

As stressed earlier, if the tests have no bearing on the treatment and are being done merely to gain extra information or to confirm a diagnosis that is already established, then you have a right to refuse to submit to a procedure. (There are times, however, when confirmation of what is suspected is necessary, but this is different from doing added tests simply to back up what is already known.) Patients often are too intimidated to question their doctors. Fortunately this is changing, but many patients still are unsure of what to do. After all, they may reason, isn't the doctor the expert? How do I know what treatment is good or bad; how can I question his (or her) judgment? On one level this is correct, but questioning can be done in an inoffensive way. After all, it is your health and your money that are at stake. The better informed you are, the more likely you are to get the kind of medical attention you need. You would be surprised at how many times a doctor will respond by saying, "Well, maybe we could wait and see how you respond to this first treatment before we get into more extensive testing."

If you get the feeling that every time you burp or have heartburn, you'll end up with stomach X rays or some other procedure, or that if you complain of an ache in the chest, you'll end up having X rays of your coronary arteries, then maybe you're being overtreated. Your doctor may be too aggressive and too procedure-oriented or too concerned about malpractice or economics. Whatever the reason, you might wish to seek out another doctor. After all, most belching or heartburn clears with simple measures over a short time, and chest pain can usually be diagnosed without high-tech tests. In most cases, little is lost by waiting and observing. Certainly, in the case of hypertension, judgment and a low-key approach produce good results in the majority of cases. Of course, if a symptom is acute or severe, especially if it is chest pain, or if it doesn't go away or gets worse, the use of additional diagnostic procedures may make a real difference in your treatment.

The following are some simple approaches that your doctor can use, in most instances, to determine whether or not there has been target-organ damage.

EYE EXAMINATION

The eyes should be one of the first organs a doctor examines during a medical checkup, especially if a patient has high blood pressure. This examination is not to check vision but to examine the condition of the blood vessels in the eyes. By shining a light into the eye, the doctor can actually see the tiny blood vessels that stretch across the retina (the "screen" in the back of the eye), and early damage to the arteries may be detected. For example, there may be tiny hemorrhages or yellow spots on the retina, indicating a lack of adequate circulation to the screen. If the arteries in the eyes are narrowed (signs of arteriosclerosis), there's a good chance that vessels elsewhere in the body may also be affected.

CHECKING OF PULSES AND HEART

Early impairment of the peripheral or surface circulation usually can be detected simply by feeling certain pulses. It is rarely necessary to undergo special circulation studies. The pulses behind the ankle or on top of the foot should be carefully checked; a weak or absent pulse in these areas indicates impaired circulation of the lower legs. The femoral arteries, which carry blood to the lower extremities, should be felt in the groin. Similarly, pulses and sounds of the carotid artery can be checked by palpating and using a stethoscope. The left lateral part of the chest can be palpated to determine whether or not the heart is enlarged, and by listening, a physician can determine whether any of the heart valves are abnormal.

ELECTROCARDIOGRAPHIC EXAMINATION

An electrocardiogram (ECG) maps the heart's electrical activity and is a standard part of any cardiovascular examination. The ECG usually reveals signs of an enlarged heart if it is present. In fact, it can detect an enlarged heart before it shows up on a chest X ray. There are instances, however, in which an electrocardiogram will not detect an enlarged left ventricle as readily as will an echocardiogram, which is a sonar or sound mapping of the heart walls and the interior of the heart. In my opinion, this increased ability to pick up early heart enlargement does not justify making echocardiography a part of the routine work-up of hypertensive patients, as is now advocated by a growing number of physicians (also see Chapter 2). This is an example of how important it is to ask how a test will change treatment. For example, my approach to treatment for a patient with mild to moderate hypertension is the same whether or not there is an enlarged heart. We treat and lower blood pressure regardless of evidence of target-organ change. If, however, a routine ECG shows evidence of cardiac enlargement, treatment may be pursued more vigorously.

An echocardiogram may be justified and useful when there are questions about the function of a heart valve and the overall function of the heart, but these are unusual situations. If all of us followed the suggestions of some physicians and performed routine echocardiograms in even five million of the forty plus million hypertensives, we would add more than one billion dollars to the cost of care. In my opinion, the majority of these patients would derive very little benefit. Echocardiography is an exciting diagnostic procedure which is extremely useful in some circumstances, but it is widely overused.

EXERCISE TOLERANCE OR STRESS TESTS

This is still another procedure that has become a routine part of a physical examination in some areas of the country, often without justification. There is no need to subject a healthy, asymptomatic person to an exercise test just because he or she happens to be over thirty-five or forty years of age. The rationale is that an exercise test can detect early changes in the coronary arteries, but as noted earlier, the large number of false positive results may lead to even more expensive and potentially dangerous tests. One example that comes to mind involved a forty-one-year-old man who came to my office a few years ago and recounted a long tale that began when he turned on a television health show. The show's medical expert advised that all men over the age of forty undergo an exercise test, especially if they had any risk factors for heart disease, such as a high blood pressure (which he had). He saw his doctor, who agreed to the procedure.

The exercise stress test measures a person's ability to walk on a treadmill at increasing speeds (up to four or more miles an hour) on a grade (compared with a hill at a 12 to 15 percent incline) for about ten to fifteen minutes. The objective is to increase the heart rate from a resting level of about 60 to 70 beats per minute to a predetermined rate of 125 to 150 beats per minute (depending on age). If the blood supply to the heart muscle is adequate at the rapid heart rate, no unusual rhythm changes or abnormalities will be noted on the ECG. Unfortunately for this man, after twelve minutes his heart rate became chaotic, and he suffered a cardiac arrest. He was revived and then hospitalized for several days, during which time he underwent even more tests, including a coronary angiography. All the tests were normal, so he was finally discharged—with a bill for more than four thousand dollars and considerable anxiety over the state of his health.

No one ever figured out why this happened. Fortunately this is a rare occurrence, but this individual never should have had the exercise stress test in the first place. His doctor should have taken the time to explain that TV newscasters haven't had much practical experience in medicine and that they usually summarize what has been reported in a medical journal or news conference without the ability to critique the usefulness of the reported procedure or treatment. Had he done this, I'm fairly certain that my new patient would not have had his "routine" test.

It also should be remembered that suggestions for "routine" testing often come from physicians at centers involved in doing procedures. It might be expected that a doctor who works all day doing echocardiograms or stress tests would believe that everyone should have one. Yet although this approach does not necessarily represent good medical care; it certainly represents expensive care. *More is not necessarily better in delivering quality care.*

There *are* indications for stress tests—the presence of unusual chest pain, the desire to determine how severe coronary artery disease is, and so on—but routine stress testing in people with hypertension is not one of them. People who have enlarged hearts and high blood pressure may have abnormal stress tests *without* the presence of coronary disease. False positives are more frequent in these individuals.

Keeping Everything in Perspective

In this chapter I have focused on the serious consequences of *uncontrolled* high blood pressure. The intent has not been to frighten but rather to reemphasize the fact that most of these consequences can be prevented or minimized by early detection and effective treatment of high blood pressure.

Hypertension *is* a serious disease, but we now have the means to diagnose it easily. In the majority of cases, elaborate and expensive work-ups are not needed and, indeed, may be counterproductive. Once hypertension has been diagnosed, an effective treatment program can almost always be devised.

Myths and Facts

MYTH: Once there is evidence of heart enlargement or kidney damage in a person with hypertension, treatment may not be effective in preventing future trouble.

FACT: Quite the contrary, lowering blood pressure may actually reduce an enlarged heart to normal size and also stop the progression of kidney disease.

MYTH: In order to obtain an accurate picture of what's going on, physicians may have to do ambulatory blood pressure monitoring, exercise stress tests, or echocardiograms on their patients with hypertension.

FACT: Nothing could be further from the truth. In the vast majority of cases none of these procedures is necessary. An accurate diagnosis can be made without the use of these tests. If we are to stop the *abuse* of technology in medicine, we must begin to use these new procedures more selectively. Patients can play a role in limiting their use by asking, "Why?" and, "How are the results going to help *me*?"

Summing Up

- Hypertension affects almost all the arteries of the body.

- Long-standing high blood pressure damages artery walls and the cells that form their surface lining. Such damage may result in hardening of the arteries or a weakening of the artery walls.

- Although hypertension is not *the* major factor responsible for angina or poor circulation, it is an important risk factor for early arteriosclerosis, which contributes to these conditions.

- Chronic high blood pressure can lead to an enlarged heart.

- *Untreated* high blood pressure can damage the filtering system of the kidneys and lead to kidney failure.

- The blood vessels carrying blood to the brain are damaged in the same way by chronic hypertension as other vessels.

- Many strokes and heart attacks are prevented each year as the result of better treatment of high blood pressure.

4

WHO SHOULD TREAT YOUR HIGH BLOOD PRESSURE?

In the good old days most of us had a family doctor who tended to most or all of our medical needs—everything from childbirth to death. Today, in an era of medical specialization, the family physician is all but extinct. The establishment of HMOs, PGPs, IPAs, DRGs, and other programs have made health care seem more like alphabet soup than the process of seeing to the needs of patients.

To complicate matters further, advertising and public relations agencies are now helping you find the right doctor or the most "humane and up-to-date hospital." Hospitals, prepaid plans, and individual physicians are competing for patients, especially patients who can pay the skyrocketing costs of modern health care.

Wherever there is competition, advertising becomes involved. In the past it was considered unethical for physicians to advertise their services, and those who stooped to such tactics were considered charlatans. Now physicians make television commercials, take out full-page ads in newspapers, rent billboards, and use subtle public relations strategies to attract patients. Some of today's health care advertising makes yesterday's snake-oil salesman seem downright respectable. Little wonder so many people have no idea where to turn for reliable health care. Should they rely on ads for "the hernia center where our board-certified specialists do hundreds or even thousands of these operations a year"? Or should they put themselves in the hands of a "sensitive, compassionate board-certified plastic surgeon" who promises a new face, tummy, or bust—*provided* that there is a certified check up front? Alternatively, should they just look in the phone book and guess?

Of course, the people who stand to lose the most by all the hoopla and advertising are the patients themselves, who bear the cost of ad campaigns by paying higher fees. Consumers should also realize that ethical, qualified physicians are probably not the ones engaging in these advertising campaigns.

Growing numbers of people find themselves trapped in a health care maze that does not meet their needs. Especially vulnerable to the pitfalls of the maze are people with chronic diseases like hypertension that require periodic checkups. It's important to have a physician who knows your medical history, can tend to your ongoing care, and can serve as your advocate in dealing with an increasingly complex health care system. In addition, a physician can help you put into perspective the media hype for new tests and treatments. But where do you go to find such a physician?

If you already have a family physician—preferably an internist or doctor trained in family practice medicine—chances are that he or she can treat your high blood pressure quite effectively. If you don't have a regular physician—and large numbers of Americans don't—then it is important that you find one. This is not always easy. There is no single formula for choosing the right doctor, but I can offer some general guidelines.

• *Decide what kind of doctor you want.* The best choice is probably an internist or a family physician with an interest in hypertension. You are unlikely to need a superspecialist or "world-renowned" researcher. In fact, you are probably better off with a competent, well-trained doctor who devotes most of his or her efforts to patient care. Pure researchers and academic specialists can be called upon in special situations, but for day-to-day routine treatment of high blood pressure, they may not be your best choice because they may not be used to or interested in uncomplicated medical problems. Recently trained cardiologists will also know how to treat hypertension, but many of them are far more interested in echocardiography, ECG monitoring, cardiac catheterization, and other new technologies than in routine patient care.

• *Check his or her credentials.* Your local medical society can provide you with a list of qualified physicians in your area. Other sources of names include the local health department, your company's medical directory, friends, or physician acquaintances. Once you have several names, you can do further checking at your local library. Physician directories published by the American Medical Association or the *Directory of Medical Specialists* provide useful background information, such as where a doctor attended medical school, year of graduation, place of training, board certification, specialty, and hospital affiliation. This may not give you a true picture of what the doctor is like, but it sets the stage for your next step.

• *Call his or her office for more information.* You can learn a good deal about a doctor and his or her general approach to patients through a simple telephone call. Start by identifying yourself; say you are looking for a regular physician and would like some preliminary information about Dr. X. Are you treated with respect and courtesy or put off with a curt "make an appointment" or "call back later"? Specific questions you should ask include:

Is the doctor seeing new patients?

What kind of practice does he or she have (solo, group, etc.)?

What are the charges for a routine office visit? Does he or she accept insurance or Medicare assignments?

What are the office hours, and who covers for him or her at other times?

What are the doctor's hospital affiliations? Is one of the hospitals convenient to you, and is it one that you would find acceptable should the need arise?

The answers will give you an idea of whether or not you see eye to eye on these nonmedical but important issues.

If you have a good feeling from your preliminary inquiries, your next step should be to make an appointment. This visit usually includes an examination. A few doctors welcome a preliminary get-acquainted session in which you can ask each other questions and decide whether or not you're likely to develop a workable physician-patient relationship. Most prefer, however, to combine this initial meeting with a medical examination, which includes asking questions about your past health history and doing a general physical examination. During this session you should not hesitate to ask as well as answer questions. Specific questions you should have in mind as the visit progresses include:

Do you communicate well with each other? Does the doctor seem interested in listening to you? Do you have his or her full attention, or does the doctor seem distracted? Are your questions answered in language you can understand?

Does the doctor seem interested in preventive care? For example, are you asked about tobacco and alcohol use, exercise, diet, or medications you may be taking?

What is his or her approach to testing and procedures? For example, does the doctor advise elaborate testing before he or she even evaluates routine measurements and laboratory tests? There should be no need for extensive X rays, exercise stress testing, elaborate kidney function tests, and such unless clearly indicated by the results of routine testing or unless you have an obviously serious or unusual problem.

Does the doctor outline what he or she expects of you? Health care is a two-way partnership, and a physician should make clear what your role will be. Be wary of a doctor who tosses off your questions or suggestions with "Just leave it to me."

Some patients expect more than doctoring from their physicians. They may want a health educator, a sympathetic ear, a person who will take time to listen and evaluate. Others may want an action-oriented physician who will do whatever is needed to fix the problem as quickly as possible without a lot of discussion. You have to decide what your particular needs are.

Of course, the selection of a primary care physician does not necessarily mean an end to your evaluation process. Generally, if you come away from your initial visit with a good feeling, you should be able to establish a satisfactory, long-term physician-patient relationship. But first impressions may be misleading. As time goes on, if you think that your care is inadequate or, conversely, that you are being overtreated or shunted off for lots of consultations without adequate cause, you may want to start all over. This is a hard thing to do, and fortunately it is not often necessary.

Alternatives to Private Individual Physicians or Groups

Increasingly, prepaid group practices like HMOs (health maintenance organizations) are taking the place of private physicians. Sometimes these plans allow you to select a physician who oversees your care; others dictate that you see whoever is available in the group. More and more, individuals may not have much choice in who provides their health care, especially if it is paid for by an employer or other third party. To keep costs in check, many large employers are switching to HMOs or other prepaid plans. There are advantages to many of these plans—they provide comprehensive care at reduced costs—but there also are disadvantages.

Without a physician to serve as your advocate in dealing with the system, you must be prepared to know and defend your own point of view. You also may have to assume more responsibility for your own medical record keeping. There may not be as much attention to follow-up and continuing care. On the plus side, however, many of these groups stress prevention and self-care which are more economical than procedure-oriented medicine—areas of high income for private physicians.

What to Expect from the Doctor Treating Your High Blood Pressure

Let's assume that you have found the right doctor or medical group to treat your high blood pressure. Just what should you expect in the way of care? Obviously the specific details depend upon the severity of your hypertension and the ease with which it is controlled. These are discussed in the following chapters. The most important thing to expect is that your blood pressure will be lowered and maintained at levels of 140/90 or below. Here is the outline of a standard approach and some criteria you can use to judge whether your own care is appropriate.

DIAGNOSIS

As stressed earlier and contrary to some opinions, you don't need to see a doctor a half dozen or more times or undergo twenty-four-hour monitoring, stress testing, and other time-consuming, expensive procedures to establish an accurate diagnosis. (See Chapter 2). A diagnosis and an adequate initial evaluation can be done in two or at the most three visits, usually two or three months apart. (Very high blood pressure can be diagnosed in a single visit.) Simple blood pressure measurements taken in the office, a physical examination, careful medical history, and routine blood and urine tests plus an electrocardiogram are usually all that's needed.

INITIAL FOLLOW-UP

Once a diagnosis is established, if the blood pressure is only slightly elevated, nondrug treatments will probably be tried for three to six months. Exceptions are cases in which the blood pressure is high (above 155–160/105–110) or where there is clear evidence of complications, such as an enlarged heart or kidney damage. During this trial period you should probably be checked after two or three months to see if there has been an improvement or a worsening of the high blood pressure.

If there is no improvement at the end of about four to six months, and blood pressures remain above 140/90, drug therapy will probably be initiated. Depending upon the severity of the hypertension and types of drugs needed, two or three follow-up visits over three to six months are usually adequate to establish the proper dosage and stabilize the blood pressure. If your hypertension is severe or if there are complications, you may be seen at monthly intervals or even every two or three weeks until your blood pressure is controlled.

LONG-TERM FOLLOW-UP

Once blood pressure is under control, most patients need to see their doctors only every four to six months or so.

Of course, there are situations in which pressure is difficult to control or in which certain medications cause adverse reactions and have to be changed every month or so. In such instances it may be necessary to see your doctor more often, but in my experience only about 15 percent of patients fall into this category. For the vast majority of people with high blood pressure, treatment is straightforward and does not require monthly or semi-monthly visits to the physician. If your pressure is controlled and your physician still insists on monthly visits, you may have the wrong doctor. If pressure isn't controlled at levels below 140/90 (most of the time) after a suitable period of time and after several attempts to find the right combination of medicine, it may be time to see a specialist in high blood pressure. About one in ten patients does not achieve normal blood pressure levels regardless of the doctor or medications used, and such a patient may have to settle for less than perfect control.

Other Health Care Personnel

Sometimes patients can benefit by seeing a dietitian, nurse educator, or other health care professional. Before making appointments with various allied health workers, ask what you can expect to gain from these visits. If you need to lose weight or reduce your sodium intake and have no idea where to begin, a dietitian can be helpful, but your physician should be able to start you on your way. If you want to give it a try on your own with the guidance of sound information, there is no compelling reason for you to rush off to your local diet center or to engage a nutrition counselor. The same is true of an exercise physiologist or health club membership. Most people can condition themselves on their own with a graduated walking program and some simple calisthenics; they don't really need extensive muscle, strength, and coordination evaluations, fancy exercise equipment, or a health club membership. In other words, most people with high blood pressure do not need an entire staff of people to help them get in shape and get their pressures down.

Alternative Therapies

The media has given considerable attention to biofeedback training, wonder diets, meditation, and other alternative treatments for high blood pressure. Some of these may produce temporary benefits, but there is little scientific evidence to support widespread claims of hypertension cures via these alternative therapies. So don't run off and sign up for the local transcendental meditation course just because the ad tempted you. Weight loss, sodium restriction, and moderate exercise do have an important role in treating high blood pressure, but the same cannot be said for faddist diets. There may be some initial improvement on such regimens, but no data as yet show that it lasts for any length of time. In Chapter 8 we will discuss the pros and cons and results of the nonpharmacologic methods of treating high blood pressure, including the use of so-called miracle diets.

It is natural to want to take control of your own destiny, and for this reason someone who claims that your blood pressure can be controlled without drugs or reliance on the medical establishment may capture your attention. Unfortunately the majority of these alternative treatments benefit their purveyors' pocketbooks more than they help the unwitting consumers. Each year Americans spend more than ten billion dollars on worthless, unproved remedies. Don't become one of those who are victimized. Rather than succumb to the ranks of the taken, it is far better for you to become a knowledgeable and discriminating consumer of legitimate medical practices.

It is a disservice to the public for responsible publications to advise that mild hypertension is really not too serious and that treatment without medication is usually all that is needed.

Summing Up

• Just because you see a doctor and take medication does not mean that your hypertension is being adequately treated. Make certain that your pressures are at or near normal.

- Don't hesitate to ask your doctor questions. The questions that you ask may serve as a catalyst toward making some necessary changes in your treatment program.

- If your doctor does not believe in treating mild to moderate hypertension, you should consider selecting a new physician who will help lower your pressures to normal levels.

5

THE ROLE OF DIET

The possible link between a high salt intake and blood pressure, as well as the fact that being heavy or obese increases your chances of having high blood pressure, diabetes, and heart disease, was discussed in Chapter 1. It would seem logical to assume that cutting down on salt in the diet and losing weight, if you are heavy, would be an effective way to lower blood pressure and reduce your risk for a heart attack. Indeed, diet is our oldest treatment for high blood pressure. But the question remains, does diet alone lower blood pressure?

As early as 1904 two French physicians recognized that blood pressure could be lowered by restricting sodium, a finding that was documented by other researchers both in the United States and abroad during the next few decades. In the 1940's, Dr. Walter Kempner at Duke University Medical Center became famous for his rice and fruit diet, a diet that restricted food intake to bowls of rice and fruit juices. This diet was originally used to treat massively obese patients, but when Dr. Kempner and his colleagues noted that it also lowered high blood pressure, they started using it to treat patients with severe hypertension. Many of these patients had already developed heart and kidney complications. While they were on the diet, marked reductions in blood pressure were noticed and kidney and heart conditions also improved. But though the diet helped, it was boring, was much too rigid for most people to follow, and was viewed by patients as akin to punishment. It was, however, one of the only treatments available at that time. In the late 1940's I had a few patients on this minimalist diet with temporary good results, but they were miserable. They stayed on it for a while because the alternatives were even more unappealing: more severe disease and often death.

Over the years a number of studies have documented that reduced sodium intake can help lower blood pressure in some people whose hypertension is associated with sodium sensitivity; in some patients with mild to moderate hypertension, weight loss can bring pressure readings back to normal. There are, of course, other health benefits associated with maintaining normal weight. People who are thin tend to have fewer heart attacks, lower blood cholesterol levels, and a lower incidence of diabetes than their overweight peers. But despite well-documented benefits of diet in at least some hypertensive patients, dietary treatment has faded into the background with the development of effective medications to lower blood pressure. Doctors know only too well that it is easier to get people to take pills every day than it is to change their eating habits radically. After all, who wants to subsist on a limited-calorie, tasteless diet when we have such an abundance of interesting and good-tasting food to tempt us? Obviously, if there is some other course available, it's only human nature to take it.

Recently there has been a renewed interest in diet as an important component in the overall approach to lowering high blood pressure. In the last fifteen or twenty years Americans have become more conscious of the part nutrition plays in maintaining good health and more adept at making low-calorie, low-salt diets palatable.

Today's dietary approach is also much more relaxed than that of the past. We now know that it is not necessary—indeed, we recognize that it is probably counterproductive and maybe even injurious to good health*—to go on an extremely restricted diet for any length of time. Any diet that omits entire classes of nutrients and does not include adequate calories and variety to maintain good nutrition should be avoided. Crash or fad diets may produce short-term results, but experience has shown that a very high percentage of the people who follow them revert to their former eating habits and are soon back where they started. *If the first miracle diet to lower blood pressure, reduce weight, and cure diabetes was truly a miracle, we would still be using it.* The truth is that most of these crash diets last about as long as it takes their sponsors to become rich and famous. In just about this much time people find out that the miracle diet hasn't produced a miracle: They're getting sick from the diet, they are unable to follow it, or it simply doesn't work.

In this chapter I will outline a commonsense dietary approach that seems to work well for my patients. In fact, many voice skepticism in the beginning that an eating program which allows them to enjoy their favorite foods without feeling starved all the time can really work. They have been led to believe that any good diet must have a strong element of self-denial. Of course, these "good" diets are doomed from the beginning. I recall one patient who illustrates a typical course.

This patient, S. G. was about 40 pounds overweight (165 pounds and five feet four inches tall). When she came to me, she had mild high blood pressure, 145/95 mmHg. A year or so earlier her family doctor had told her she must lose weight and also cut down on her salt intake because of her blood pressure. He had given her a printed diet sheet and a list of salty foods to avoid.

For S. G. the diet represented a special sacrifice. Good food was very important to her; cooking and entertaining were favorite pastimes. The diet plan allowed her about 1,000 calories a day and, although balanced, was unimaginative and limited in its food choices. She could immediately see it left little room for her flair for preparing food—to say nothing of her enjoyment of eating it. But she wanted to lose the excess weight, and she was concerned about her blood pressure, so she gave the diet a chance.

She stuck to it faithfully for a few weeks and lost seven or eight pounds. Then her son came home from college for summer vacation, and before long she was back in her old groove of cooking her family's favorite foods. At first she tried watching them enjoy things like imaginative pasta dishes, pork chops, and her special pastries and cookies while she nibbled at steamed vegetables, bland chicken, and fresh fruit. It wasn't long before she succumbed to the kinds of food she had enjoyed most of her life.

"I knew I wasn't doing what I was supposed to," she told me, "and I felt guilty every time I went back to my family doctor. I decided I'd take the summer off, and go back on the diet when my son returned to college." But then the holidays rolled around, and again the diet went out the window. "I stopped going to the doctor altogether," she confessed, "he always seemed to be disappointed in me, I felt more and more guilty, and I must admit, our once good relationship deteriorated rapidly." But when her gynecologist found her blood pressure was too high, she became worried enough to start anew.

Her story had a familiar ring and reinforced my contention that a diet based on denial and guilt simply doesn't work for most people. The litany of excuses from patients on why they can't adhere to a diet is amusing but sad. It always starts with "But, Doctor, I really don't eat very much. Let me tell you what I had for breakfast. . . ." Even more important, I know that in most instances it's both unrealistic and unnecessary to expect people to forgo favorite foods and throw out lifelong eating habits. Instead of putting S. G. on yet another regimen, I enlisted the aid of a dietitian who works with overweight patients to come up with an eating plan that included some of her favorite foods. I also carefully reviewed with her the diet that I have been using for many years which was low in salt and fat but was varied and palatable. The patient was encouraged to walk for a half hour every day. I told our frustrated patient that we would try three months on this more varied but low-calorie diet to see whether it had a beneficial effect on her blood pressure. When she came to see me at the end of that time, she obviously was much happier, with both herself and her treatment program. "I don't even feel I'm on a diet," she said. "But just look at me—I've lost twelve pounds, and I'm a full dress size smaller!"

Her blood pressure, although still in a borderline area, was lower than on my previous examination. I told her to continue on her regimen for another three months, and then we would decide whether she should go on medication to lower her blood pressure even more. At the end of another three months she had lost eight more pounds and was just as enthusiastic as before. "I'm back to a size twelve," she boasted, and her blood pressure was almost normal. I saw no reason to start medication at this point, especially since she was continuing her steady weight loss.

That was more than a year ago. Her blood pressure is now in the normal range, and more than thirty pounds have been lost and kept off. More important, S. G. now knows that she can still prepare and enjoy gourmet meals and, at the same time, keep her weight under control. She has learned to modify her eating habits to reduce portion size; she also has discovered that dishes can be flavored with a variety of spices, herbs, and complementary foods without even touching her salt shaker. Later I'll review the basic principles of a low-calorie, nutritious, and varied diet that you can stay on and enjoy.

Someday this patient may need to take medication, but for the time being, she is doing well without it. Her blood cholesterol has also dropped since I first saw her, and she enjoys her renewed feelings of success and high self-esteem.

Not every hypertensive patient can be treated by relatively simple life-style changes as successfully as S. G. was. In fact, the majority cannot. But even those who do need medication often can reduce their dosages, and consequently the cost of treatment and chances of side effects, by following a commonsense program of modifying their eating habits.

As noted earlier, in beginning the treatment of high blood pressure, it is important to try the nondrug approach before starting medication, especially for people with mild to moderate hypertension. There is no doubt that lowering blood pressure with diet and exercise is preferable to prescribing drugs, and a fair trial of three to six months is the only way to know whether this approach will work. If initial pressures are very high, however, it may be prudent to start medication *and* dietary changes at the same time. If pressures come down to normal and weight loss and sodium restriction have been accomplished, medication can be reduced or withdrawn later to see whether or not pressures remain at normal levels.

Role of Diet

The precise role of diet in the development of high blood pressure is unknown and varies from person to person. In general, two components—excessive weight and sodium—are known to contribute to high blood pressure in people with a genetic predisposition to develop the disease. It should be noted, however, that there are people of normal weight who become hypertensive, and conversely, there are plenty of overweight people with normal pressures. The same goes for sodium: Some people can eat huge amounts of salt (the most common dietary source of sodium) and still have normal blood pressure, while others who consume very little have hypertension. It is frustrating to have a friend or relative who may gorge him or herself with ice cream and heavily salted foods remain thin and have normal blood pressure and cholesterol levels, while all you may have to do is seemingly look at a salt shaker or an egg and your blood pressure and cholesterol rise. But then again, that's what heredity and genes are all about. Some population studies indicate that other dietary elements, like potassium and calcium, may protect against high blood pressure, but this has not been proved.

The typical American diet tends to be high in calories, cholesterol, saturated fat, and sugar or other refined sweeteners. On the positive side, we consume a wide variety of foods, and nutritional deficiencies are very rare. In recent years all of us have become more nutrition-conscious and have made substantial changes in our diets. We are eating less bacon, eggs, butter, red meats, and other sources of saturated animal fats. We are eating more pasta and other complex starches and dietary fiber.

We are more conscious of the role that cholesterol and sodium play in our futures.

All these changes are good, but with them have come some problems. Americans tend to look for quick fixes, and this often means turning to a fad diet, unnecessary supplements, or an unproved remedy. Every six to twelve months yet another miracle diet hits the best-seller list. The Bloomingdales, California, Rockefeller, and any number of other diets have come and gone. Some of these diet schemes are fairly reasonable, but others, such as the Immune Power, Drinking Man's, Atkins, Scarsdale, Cambridge, and Beverly Hills, may promote serious nutritional imbalances and, in some instances, can be quite dangerous. The same may be said for the currently popular liquid protein diets that may work well in getting off those first fifteen or twenty pounds but that most people just can't (and shouldn't) stay on. Not only may they be dangerous, but also the dieters learn nothing about good long-term eating habits. These diets should not be recommended in programs of long-term care for hypertensive patients despite reports that blood pressure is lowered when they are used. In "malignant obesity," where a person is more than sixty to seventy pounds overweight, a crash diet with a protein mix might be acceptable for several weeks as a starter, but a balanced low-calorie diet should be substituted after this time.

Many food manufacturers are also quick to take advantage of our dietary insecurities. In recent years the supermarket shelves have been flooded by a mind-boggling assortment of "lite" products. Unfortunately there is no standard definition of "lite." Some of these foods are low in sodium, fat, sugar, or other ingredients that the public perceives of as being detrimental. Others, such as some of the "lite" oils, are merely lighter in color or flavor than the standard varieties. It's little wonder many people are thoroughly confused.

People believe that "natural" foods, presumably chemical-free, are healthier than foods grown with the benefit of artificial fertilizers and pesticides or those containing additives or preservatives. The facts do not bear out these misconceptions. All foods, indeed, all living matter, are composed of chemicals. Granted, some chemicals—including some that occur naturally in foods—are dangerous, but many others are essential to maintain life. There is no evidence that foods grown with "natural" fertilizers are more nutritious than those grown with artificial fertilizers. Moreover, some additives serve only cosmetic purposes and could be eliminated from foods, but others are essential to preserve nutrients and to retard the growth of harmful bacteria or molds.

Of course, some of these factors may not have a direct relationship to our central concern here—namely, high blood pressure and other risk factors for heart disease—but they are relevant to the basic theme of using common sense to control a serious health problem. Perhaps more than any other life-style factor, diet should be governed by moderation and common sense. The success story of the patient I just told about, S. G., is a prime example: For her, and for millions of other average Americans, a dietary regimen that ignores personal food preferences and asks for an abrupt change in lifelong eating habits simply doesn't work over the long term. A commonsense approach that takes into account what you now eat and then shows how you can modify it *will* succeed.

This doesn't happen automatically. You do have to

take a careful look at what you eat and pay attention to problem areas. One of the best ways to determine exactly what you eat in the course of a day is to keep a food diary for a week or two. In my experience, most overweight patients are convinced that they are not overeating. When they list their intakes for a few days, however, it is easy to spot high-calorie foods that are consumed almost unconsciously: the nuts or chips served with cocktails or munched while they watch TV; the several glasses of soft drinks or juice consumed instead of water over the course of a day; the glass or two of wine or beer; the bacon bits, cheese dressing, and other high-calorie salad toppings, to mention only a few. Even small amounts of these items can add hundreds of extra calories. If analysis of a food diary shows that you are consuming, say, 400 calories a day in such items, you can lose three to four pounds a month simply by eliminating them or substituting low-calorie counterparts.

The rule is that you can lose a pound of weight if you burn up 3,500 more calories than you take in. Thus, if you cut your intake by 500 calories a day, you will lose about one pound a week (500 × 7 = 3,500 calories, or one pound).

I have also come to believe that exercise helps burn up more calories than we are told (see the chart in Chapter 6 listing various activities and amount of calories they consume). Often patients will lose more weight by exercising than they are supposed to according to the charts. For example, the 300 to 350 calories a week used up by playing tennis for one hour or the 180 calories an hour burned up by walking shouldn't result in any significant weight loss, but the exercise seems to do so in some people. This may be related to a change in certain metabolic processes, actual absorption of food, or other factors that we know little about.

Reductions in portion size is the best way to reduce calories without depriving yourself of favorite foods. I instruct patients to start any diet by cutting portions in half and limiting the cakes, candies, cookies, and bread to a greater degree than fruits, vegetables, and other high-nutrition, low-calorie foods. The foods that people like are not restricted or eliminated; just the amounts are. For example, if someone really loves a good steak once in a while, that's okay. But it should be a three- or four-ounce fillet, not a twelve-ounce sirloin. Good advice to the person in the family who shops would be to buy less. Serve two or three chicken breasts for two people instead of four or five, and cook eight to twelve ounces of fish instead of a pound or more. Most of us eat everything we're given, so if we're presented with less, we'll eat less. If there are teenagers in the household, they do need more food than older people to support their growth, but most of us consume more than we actually need.

For an adult to reduce his or her calorie intake by 500 to 800 calories a day is not too difficult. If 200 more calories a day are used up by extra walking, that also helps. With a little imagination, chances are you can find easy ways to cut your food intake without turning your household into a diet kitchen. (See the accompanying Tips to Cut Calories.) A few examples of daily menus with foods that are low in salt and fat content appear at the end of this chapter.

The Question of Metabolism

Many of my overweight patients maintain that they do not overeat; instead, they insist that something is wrong with their metabolism. Yet in these people the standard tests for thyroid function as a mirror of metabolic rate are usually normal. Recent scientific studies, however, support their contention to a degree. Increasingly, researchers are finding that overweight people do have a genetic predisposition to metabolize food more efficiently than their slender counterparts. They actually require less food for their day-to-day activities, and the excess is stored as body fat. This does not mean, however, that they are doomed to be fat. Increased physical activity, coupled with a moderate decrease in food intake, will help maintain ideal weight. Obese people also have more fat cells that pick up and store fat. These cells are formed mostly during childhood or adolescence. This is why it is important not to overfeed young people. *The prediction that a fat child or adolescent will become a fat adult is true more often than not.*

Repeated starvation or crash diets also can alter your metabolic rate. When you go on an extreme low-calorie diet, your body reacts just as it would if you were really starving. Your metabolic rate slows down to conserve as much energy as possible. After a time this will be reset at a lower, more efficient point. When you resume eating a normal diet, your metabolism—the rate at which you burn up calories—will not necessarily be able to return to its prediet state. Consequently, you will not be able to eat as much as before without gaining weight. A sensible eating program that allows a slow, steady weight loss of a pound or two a week, along with increased physical activity, will minimize the chances of altering basic metabolism. Even if, in your case, this program does not result in a lowering of blood pressure, it *will* make you feel and look better and will certainly help reduce your risks of a heart attack or diabetes.

Benefits of Weight Loss

As stressed earlier, weight loss does not always bring blood pressure down to normal levels, but many hypertensive patients who lose at least some excess weight will also achieve reduced blood pressure. For example, Dr. E. Reisin, who is now in New Orleans, studied the effects of weight reduction in eighty-one hypertensive patients. All the participants lost at least 3 kilograms (6.6 pounds), and seventy-three lost more than 5 kilograms (11 pounds). All but two showed a meaningful reduction in blood pressure; 75 percent of those who were not on antihypertensive medication achieved normal pressures. In a group of patients whose blood pressures were not controlled by drugs alone, 61 percent achieved normal readings with weight reduction and medication. Other studies have not shown such good results, and it is difficult to predict when or if weight loss will work; but it can't hurt and is worth a try if it's attempted in a sensible fashion.

The Sodium Question

Sodium intake is the other major dietary factor linked to high blood pressure, but we cannot say for certain just how important it is as a cause of hypertension. For about ten to fifteen million adult Americans who may be particularly sensitive to sodium, there is little doubt that it plays a role in high blood pressure. But this accounts for only about a third of our hypertensive population. In general, blacks tend to be more sodium sensitive than whites. Some researchers believe that

Tips to Reduce Calorie Consumption

1. Go easy on fatty foods, especially meats, cheese, butter or margarine, and foods with a high portion of hidden fat, such as creamy sauces, salad dressings, and pastries. When shopping, pick lean cuts of meat and trim fat before cooking.

2. Instead of whole milk, switch to low-fat or skim milk, especially when cooking. To get used to the taste of low-fat milk, start first with 2 percent fat, then 1 percent and finally skim. For more consistency, try adding a teaspoon of non-fat dried milk to a glass of skim. As a substitute for whipped cream, try whipping evaporated skim milk in a chilled mixing bowl. Chilled non-fat dry milk also can be whipped. Avoid nondairy creamers and nondairy toppings—these are loaded with saturated fats (palm or coconut oils) and calories.

3. The way you prepare foods also affects the calorie content. Roast, bake, broil, or simmer meat, poultry, and fish. When preparing meat in a skillet, use a nonstick pan which can tolerate a high heat. Meat should be seared quickly; then lower the heat to cook to desired doneness and drain off the fat. Better still, cook under the broiler, using a rack to let the fat drain off. Discard the drippings, or chill and then remove the solidified fat.

4. Potatoes, carrots, and other vegetables quickly absorb fat and therefore should never be browned with meat. Instead of flavoring with butter, try herbs, vegetable juices, or other low-calorie substitutes.

5. In poultry, most of the fat is stored under the skin, which should be removed before cooking. Baste with broth, wine, tomato juice, or other low-fat liquid. Avoid pre-basted turkey, which is often injected with saturated coconut oil.

6. When cooking soups, stews, chili, and other meat-based dishes, prepare in advance and then chill until the fat solidifies on the top, and can be easily removed.

7. To further reduce the fat used when making stir-fried dishes, use nonstick cookware and nonstick vegetable cooking sprays instead of oil and shortening.

8. In baking, experiment with reducing the fat. For example, you can cut the amount of fat in pie crusts by at least a third and use a little extra water to prevent crumbling.

9. Try making your own salad dressings and spreads or buy the low-calorie substitutes. Lemon juice and low-fat yogurt or cottage cheese whipped in a blender make a tasty low-calorie creamy dressing. A teaspoon of blue cheese or sprinkling of parmesan will add a cheese flavor with a fraction of the calories of commercial cheese dressings.

10. To reduce the calories in spreads, use a blender or food processor to whip cold water into butter or margarine. This is the same method food manufacturers use in making the "lite" or reduced-calorie spreads. By doing it yourself, you can save the high cost of the commercial varieties. Also, let the butter or margarine get soft before using it—it can be spread thinly and you're not as likely to use as much.

There are many more "tricks" you can use to cut calories. Once you start thinking in these terms, you'll discover many more, and will soon find you don't even miss all that extra fat.

there is a genetic basis for their increased response to sodium, but this has not been proved. The sensitivity could also be acquired through excessive consumption of salt or a decreased intake of other minerals such as potassium and calcium.

Sodium is one of several essential elements called electrolytes which are needed to maintain the proper fluid and chemical balance in the body. The kidneys are responsible for regulating the proper level of sodium in the body; they conserve sodium when levels are low and excrete it in the urine when there is an excess. Most of the time this system is extraordinarily efficient, and there are no problems. In some people, however, the kidneys are unable to handle large amounts of sodium, and as a result, the volume of fluid in the body increases. This can overload the system and cause hypertension that is dependent on the extra fluid volume. When patients with this form of volume-dependent high blood pressure are given diuretics or other medications to reduce fluid, their blood pressures come down.

In general, population groups that consume large amounts of salt have a higher incidence of hypertension than those with very low-salt diets. A medical scientist who has devoted much of his career to studying the effects of salt on high blood pressure is Dr. Lot Page. He has studied a number of population groups in nonindustrialized areas—for example, desert nomads in the Middle East and the people of the Marshall Islands in the Pacific—and has found that hypertension is very rare among them. He attributes this to their low-salt diets. In contrast, hypertension is common in many parts of Japan, the United States and other countries where diets are high in salt. In studies that I participated in, along with physicians from the University of Michigan Medical School, in the 1950s and 1960s in the West Indies and the Bahamas, where hypertension and strokes are extremely common, even on remote islands, we found that salt intake is higher than in the United States. The drinking water is high in salt, fish is often preserved by being coated with salt, and soups and other dishes are heavily salted before being served. If you have been to the Bahamas, for example, you may have experienced some ankle swelling after a few days—a sign of salt retention. Most of us can tolerate this type of a diet for a short time, but it may result in increased blood pressures in some people and could be dangerous for someone who has a poorly functioning heart.

A few researchers have found that some people with normal blood pressure will experience a definite rise when they are given large amounts of salt, either in food or intravenously, through a process called sodium loading. This is especially true for blacks as well as for some, but not all, people with borderline high blood pressure.

In contrast, many people can eat very large amounts of salt with no effect on their blood pressures. This seems to substantiate the theory that there are sodium-sensitive and sodium-resistant people. In fact, this was demonstrated years ago in laboratory animals by Dr. Lewis Dahl at the Brookhaven, New York, National Laboratory. Dr. Dahl developed strains of rats that were sodium-sensitive and also developed hypertension, and others that were sodium-resistent and never or rarely developed hypertension despite high sodium intakes. These strains of rats are now used throughout the world to study hypertension.

Among humans there is no truly accurate scientific way of determining who is sodium-sensitive or who is sodium-resistant without specific tests. Fortunately tests are not often necessary. From a practical point of view it makes sense to try sodium restriction before drug therapy to lower blood pressure is started. If there is no improvement after six to eight weeks of following a low-salt diet, it can be assumed that sodium is probably not a major factor in sustaining the high blood pressure and the next step in therapy can be undertaken. Frequently the desired reduction in the amount of salt is achieved by simple means. Sometimes all that is needed is to stop adding salt to foods in the cooking process and at the table. A good rule is first to try to cut salt intake in half, as you would the portions of food. Normally people take in about ten grams (two teaspoonfuls) of salt a day in foods and additives. *If you can cut this down to a little less than one teaspoonful (four grams) a day, you will probably see some decrease in blood pressure (if it is going to occur).* More rigid restriction might work a little better but is very difficult to achieve and follow in our world of restaurants, and processed foods. However, for people with poor heart function (heart failure) more rigid salt restriction is necessary.

When I urge my patients to cut back on salt, many argue that this will take all the taste out of food. Actually I have found that it is relatively easy to retrain taste buds to accept alternatives to salt. Indeed, researchers have determined that the taste for sodium is acquired; we are not born with it. We actually develop in a sea of salty water (the amniotic fluid) and have spent several months "drinking" this mildly salty fluid before birth. Still, newborn babies prefer sweet to salty foods and will readily accept unsalted foods. One of the ways that hypertension might be prevented in a genetically susceptible family, although there is no proof of this yet, is to keep the children on a low-salt diet from infancy on. With this in mind, some years ago many of us who were involved in hypertension research petitioned baby food manufacturers to reduce the sodium content of baby foods. The salt *was* reduced, but lo and behold, some mothers who tasted the food before giving it to their babies began to add salt so that the food tasted better. What they forgot was that their babies had not acquired their mother's taste for salt and would eat bland food if they were hungry.

SOURCES OF SODIUM

We tend to use the terms "salt" and "sodium" interchangeably. Actually sodium chloride (NaCl) is the chemical name for table salt, which is 40 percent sodium and 60 percent chloride. A teaspoon of salt contains 2.3 grams (2,300 milligrams or 0.08 ounces) of sodium. To survive, the body needs only a very small amount of sodium—about 220 milligrams (less than a quarter of a gram) a day. To be on the safe side, the adult recommended dietary allowance calls for 1.1 to 3.3 grams of sodium. Thus, the equivalent of a teaspoon of table salt per day will provide more than ample sodium for a

TABLE 5:1
General Dietary Guidelines
for People on a Low-Salt—Low-Fat Diet

This is just a guide. It does not have to be followed rigidly to maintain a reasonable low-salt diet. For example, an occasional peanut or cup of soup is okay unless you have had heart failure, which would call for a more rigid program. Foods highest in sodium are capitalized.

YOU MAY USE	USE SPARINGLY
Seasonings	
Nonsalt seasonings	Salt in cooking or at table
Milk	
Skim, low-fat, or evaporated skim milk	Buttermilk, whole milk, chocolate milk, condensed milk, instant cocoa, nondairy cream substitute, sour cream, cream, ice cream, aerosol whipped toppings, whole milk yogurt, sherbet, ice milk, creamed soups, half-and-half
Beverages	
Instant, regular, and decaffeinated coffee, tea, cocoa (plain—not with milk powder), seltzer, wine, alcoholic beverages in moderation	Commercial soft drinks

TABLE 5:1 (*continued*)

~~YOU~~ MAY USE	USE SPARINGLY
Meat, Fish, and Poultry Fresh, unsalted, all fat and skin removed; CHICKEN, turkey, FISH, VEAL; shrimp once weekly; low-sodium diet-packed salmon, shrimp, or tuna	Frozen fish fillets; canned, salted or pickled fish, such as HERRING, SMOKED SALMON, or ANCHOVIES; canned, salted, or smoked meat (BACON, bologna, FRANKS, SAUSAGE, SALT PORK, CORNED BEEF, other cold cuts). DUCK, TURKEY ROLL, HEAVILY MARBLED MEAT, skin and fat from poultry, SPARE RIBS, commercial frozen dinners, LIVER, KIDNEY. (Shellfish not more than three times weekly)
Eggs Two or three eggs weekly; egg white and substitutes	
Cheese Low-salt cottage cheese, farmer, pot cheese, skim-milk ricotta, and other low-salt and low-saturated-fat cheese	American, Swiss, muenster, cheese spreads, and all other cheeses
Fats Corn, soybean, sesame seeds, sunflower oils; unsalted polyunsaturated margarine; low-sodium mayonnaise	Butter, salted margarine, bacon fat, salt pork, meat fat, olives, products containing coconut or palm oils, lard or solid shortening, commercial salad dressings and mayonnaise, peanut butter, salted nuts

TABLE 5:1 (*continued*)

YOU MAY USE	USE SPARINGLY
Salad Dressing Lemon juice or fresh lemon, white or cider vinegar, or salt-free ketchup or salt-free chili sauce added to one of the above oils	All commercial salad dressings and mayonnaise
Breads Regular whole grain or enriched bread, unsalted melba toast, plain matzo, low-sodium bread and crackers, unsalted pretzels and mayonnaise	Salted crackers, commercial cakes, muffins, pancake mixes, etc.; salted pretzels, potato chips, popcorn, corn chips; pizza; dark rye and self-rising flour
Cereals Puffed wheat, puffed rice, shredded wheat biscuits, oatmeal, cream of wheat (not instant), Familia, muesli, wheat germ	Cooked cereals containing sodium; dried cereals other than those listed, cereals with coconut
Rice, pasta, and potatoes WITHOUT added salt, cream, or butter; WITH unsaturated vegetable oil or margarine	Creamed, scalloped, or fried in unknown fat
Vegetables All fresh or frozen except as indicated	Canned vegetables or vegetable juices, frozen peas or lima beans, sauerkraut, pickles, relish

TABLE 5:1 (*continued*)

YOU MAY USE	USE SPARINGLY
Fruit	
All fresh, canned, or frozen without preservatives; sun-dried	Maraschino cherries; canned, frozen or dried fruits which contains salt or preservatives (read labels); glazed fruit
Syrups, sugars, and candies	
Sugar, honey, pure maple syrup, pure jellies and jams, white or light brown sugar	Dark brown sugar; molasses and candies containing salt or saturated fats (read labels); coconut
Desserts	
Fruit, tapioca, rice pudding, fruit, or water ices; homemade pies, cakes, and desserts in moderation	Commercial cakes, pies, doughnuts, sweet rolls, pastries, puddings, and mixes
Other foods	
Allspice, basil, bay leaves, caraway, chives, cinnamon, curry powder, dill, garlic, ginger, prepared horseradish without salt, lemon juice, mint, mustard (dry), nutmeg, onion, oregano, paprika, parsley, pepper (black, red, and white), poppyseed, saccharin, sage, thyme, vanilla extract, vinegar, wine for flavoring (not cooking wine)	Bouillon cubes or bouillon powders, baking powder or soda, canned soups, prepared mustard, horseradish, Worcestershire sauce, soy sauce, ketchup, chili sauce, celery, onion or garlic salts, cooking wine, meat tenderizer (or MSG), tomato paste, pickled relish

TABLE 5:1 (*continued*)

YOU MAY USE	USE SPARINGLY
FAVOR FISH, VEAL, OR CHICKEN RATHER THAN RED MEATS SUCH AS STEAK OR ROAST BEEF	LIMIT INTAKE OF DAIRY PRODUCTS SUCH AS MILK, EGGS, BUTTER, AND CHEESE

Adapted from "A Sensible Low-Salt, Low-Fat Diet" by Marvin Moser, M.D.

healthy person. (The average American consumes about two teaspoonfuls of salt daily.)

On the surface you would think that it would be easy to reduce sodium intake. All you need to do is remove the salt shaker from the table, use little or no salt in preparing foods, and avoid processed foods that are high in salt. The latter is where most people run into problems. Studies have found that most of our sodium intake is hidden in processed foods, including many that do not taste at all salty—soft drinks, ice cream, breakfast cereals, bread, and commercial pastries, to name a few. Tables at the end of this chapter list foods that should be avoided by people on low-salt diets and also outline the basics of putting together a low-salt diet.

Detecting hidden sodium in processed foods is made more difficult by food labels that are often confusing or misleading. Recently the Food and Drug Administration (FDA) established uniform definitions for words used to describe sodium content. For example, if the label says a product is sodium-free, it must contain less than two hundredths of a gram or under 5 milligrams per serving. "Very low sodium" means 35 milligrams or less per serving; "low sodium" translates to 140 milligrams or less per serving. "Unsalted" simply means processed with the normal amounts of salt, while "reduced sodium" means the amount of salt used in processing has been reduced by 75 percent.

Many food flavorings, additives, and preservatives are high in sodium. (Common examples are listed in the table on high-salt foods at the end of this chapter.) Some medicines, such as antacids or laxatives containing sodium bicarbonate, sodium citrate, or sodium phosphate, also are high in sodium, *but unless you use these medications frequently, you probably are not adding much sodium to your diet.* Your pharmacist can tell you what products contain enough sodium to make a difference.

SALT SUBSTITUTES

In recent years a number of salt substitutes have been introduced. Most of these contain *potassium* chloride instead of sodium. These products can be tolerated by healthy people with normal kidneys, but they can be dangerous for those with kidney damage or for people taking potassium-sparing diuretics. Both too much and too little potassium in the blood can lead to muscle weakness and serious complications, including unusual heart rhythms. Before using a salt substitute containing potassium chloride, you should check with your doctor, and even then, use it sparingly. Many salt substitutes are bitter-tasting, and you may have to try several brands to find one that you can tolerate. It is important that the potassium level of the blood remains within reasonably normal limits, and the use of extra potassium can be important for some people on diuretics. Remember, however, that too much potassium may cause trouble.

Blends of spices and herbs are used as salt substitutes, and there is no problem with these products so long as they do not contain monosodium glutamate

TABLE 5:2
Sodium and Calorie Content of Common High-Salt Foods*

FOOD	AMOUNT	SODIUM IN MILLIGRAMS	CALORIES
Almonds (roasted and salted)	1 oz	55	176
Bacon (Canadian, broiled or fried)	1 slice	442	65
Biscuits	1 oz	185	104
Broth (canned beef or chicken)	1 cup	782	16
Bologna (beef)	1 slice	230	72
Bouillon			
Beef	1 cup	1,358	19
Chicken	1 cup	1,484	21
Carrots (canned)	8 oz	535	64
Catsup (ketchup)	1 tbp	156	16
Cheese (cheddar)	1 oz	176	114
Coffee cake (made with self-rising flour)	1 medium piece	310	232
Corn chips	1 oz	218	153
Corned beef	1 slice	294	46
Fast foods			
Big Mac	1	963	541
Vanilla shake	1	250	324

*Remember, if you are on a low-salt diet, you should probably not take in more than 2,000 milligrams of sodium a day. One pickle and a Big Mac will just about do it, leaving nothing for later on.

TABLE 5:2 (*continued*)

FOOD	AMOUNT	SODIUM IN MILLIGRAMS	CALORIES
Frankfurter (beef)	1	461	145
Ham (regular, 11% fat)	1 slice	373	52
Lima beans (canned)	8½ oz	536	41
Milk			
1% fat	1 cup	123	102
Chocolate, 1% fat	1 cup	152	158
Olives (green)	3	385	15
Oysters (canned)	3½ oz	206	76
Pancakes	1 oz	412	164
Peas (canned)	1 cup	493	150
Peanuts (roasted and salted)	1 oz	138	170
Pickle (dill, medium)	1	928	5
Pickle relish (sweet)	1 tbp	107	21
Pizza (cheese, regular crust)	¼ of 12-in crust	673	326
Potato chips (Lay's)	1 oz	260	150
Pretzel twists (hard)	10	1,010	235
Salmon (canned pink)	⅖ cup	387	141
Saltines	4 oz	123	48
Sardines (canned in oil)	4 oz	735	175
Sauerkraut (canned)	⅔ cup	666	21
Sausage (pork)	1 link	1,020	265

TABLE 5:2 (*continued*)

FOOD	AMOUNT	SODIUM IN MILLIGRAMS	CALORIES
Soups (commercially prepared)			
Chunky chicken, canned, ready to serve	1 cup	887	178
Chicken noodle, canned, made with water	1 cup	1,107	75
Chicken noodle, dry	1 cup	1,284	53
Soy sauce (La Choy)	1 tbp	975	8
Spinach (canned)	7¾ oz	519	42
Tomato juice (canned or bottled)	1 cup	878	45
Tuna (canned light in water)	6½ oz	523	184
Worcestershire sauce	1 tbp	147	12

(MSG) or other sources of sodium. There are a number of mixed blends on the market, or you can make your own (see sample recipes at the end of this chapter.) There also are a number of excellent cookbooks featuring low-salt recipes; a sample listing can be found later.

Dozens of studies have been carried out to determine whether or not high blood pressure can be lowered by restricting sodium. Most agree that a decrease of about 5 to 7 mmHg systolic and 3 to 5 mmHg diastolic can be accomplished by the kind of moderate salt restriction described here. In some cases a greater decrease in blood pressure has occurred. In others, a sodium-restricted diet was no better than a regular diet consumed by a control group.

If you start with pressures of 145/95, salt restriction may be all that is needed. If that doesn't work, don't be upset or disappointed. Simple medication will probably produce the desired results. In almost all cases some salt restriction will help make medication more effective *so that cutting down on salt intake is a good recommendation for all people with hypertension.*

In the 1950s my colleagues and I did an experiment in which a group of people with hypertension who were resistant to medication reduced their salt intakes from twelve grams a day to five grams a day. This was not too difficult to accomplish; blood pressure control was considerably improved. We then added salt pills (coded so that the subjects did not know what was being given) and got their salt intakes back up to twelve grams a day. Yes, blood pressures rose despite continuation of medication.

Other Dietary Factors

POTASSIUM

Potassium is a mineral essential to maintaining proper body chemistry. Muscles, including the heart, re-

Recipes for Spice and Herbal Salt Substitutes

HERB SEASONING

2 tbp dried dillweed or
  basil leaves, crumbled
2 tbp onion powder (not
  onion salt)
1 tsp dried oregano leaves,
  crumbled

1 tsp celery seed
¼ tsp grated dried lemon
  peel
Pinch of fresh-ground
  pepper

SPICY BLEND I

2 tbp dried savory,
  crumbled
1 tbp dry mustard
2½ tsp onion powder
(not onion salt)

1 ¼ tsp fresh ground white
  pepper
1 ¼ ground cumin
½ tsp garlic powder

1¼ tsp curry powder

SPICY BLEND II

½ tsp cayenne pepper
1 tbp garlic powder
1 tsp of each of the
  following, ground

basil
marjoram
thyme
rosemary
savory

mace
onion powder
black pepper
sage
cumin

quire specific amounts of potassium to function properly. Under normal conditions a diet that includes a variety of fruits and vegetables will provide adequate potassium. Some researchers, such as Dr. Louis Tobian at the University of Minnesota, think that potassium helps protect against high blood pressure. He cites as evidence the low incidence of high blood pressure among populations that consume a diet of mostly fruits, roots, grains, and other plant food—the kind of diet our ancestors consumed. As humankind evolved on this kind of diet—high in potassium and low in sodium—the kidneys became efficient at excreting the excess potassium and conserving sodium. Today, our diet is quite different—high in sodium and, compared with prehistoric societies, low in potassium. Dr. Tobian suggests that our physical evolution has not kept pace with our dietary changes and that by returning to a diet of mostly plant foods, we could reduce the incidence of high blood pressure.

Some recent studies suggest that people who include two or three good sources of potassium in their daily diets have a lower incidence of strokes than their counterparts whose diets are very low in potassium—again, an observation that requires further proof. It may well be that a combination of a high-sodium and low-potassium intake contributes to high blood pressure. Even in the absence of absolute scientific proof, it seems prudent to go easy on sodium and include potassium-rich foods (see the table of low-salt, high-potassium foods at the end of this chapter) in the diet. (To repeat a word of caution: If you have kidney disease, you have to be careful about potassium intake.)

Hypertensive patients on certain diuretic medications may encounter special problems related to potassium. Diuretics are prescribed to remove excess sodium and fluid from the body; in that process excessive amounts of potassium also may be washed away via the kidneys. In time this can lead to potassium depletion, resulting in muscle weakness and other symptoms. This is why doctors may periodically measure potassium levels in the blood of patients on diuretics. *Most* people, especially those under sixty years of age, can compensate for the lost potassium without problems. Some, however, such as the elderly (who may not be on a balanced diet) or patients with heart disease, may need to take potassium supplements or a medication that helps conserve potassium (for information on the potassium-sparing diuretics, see Chapter 7).

CALCIUM

There have been recent reports that calcium may play a role in blood pressure control. It may well be that a high-salt, low-calcium diet contributes to hypertension in some people, but in 1986 premature and overly enthusiastic reports in the media led many hypertensive patients to begin treating themselves with high doses of calcium pills. At this point doctors simply do not know the exact role that calcium plays. Some studies have found a lowering of blood pressure among patients put on calcium supplements, and others have found just the opposite. At present calcium pills should not be considered part of a treatment program.

Your diet should however, provide adequate calcium (the recommended dietary allowances for most adults are 800 to 1,000 milligrams per day). You should not take calcium pills unless they are specifically recommended by your doctor. Unfortunately calcium has become another diet fad; it is now being added to everything from orange juice to breakfast cereals. A diet that includes two or three servings of milk (preferably low-fat) or milk products provides enough calcium for most people. Too much calcium may cause trouble. It is quite possible that because of the recent media hype about calcium, there will be an increase in the occurrence of kidney stones within the next few years.

TABLE 5:3
Low-Salt, High-Potassium Foods

FOOD	SERVING SIZE	POTASSIUM (milligrams)	SODIUM
Apricots	3 medium	281	1
Apricots (dried)	8 halves	490	13
Asparagus	6 spears	278	2
Avocado	½ medium	604	4
Banana	1 medium	569	1
Beans (white, cooked)	½ cup	416	7
Beans (green)	1 cup	189	5
Broccoli	1 stalk	267	10
Cantaloupe	¼ medium	251	12
Carrots	2 small	341	47
Dates	10 medium	648	1
Grapefruit	½ medium	135	1
Mushrooms	4 large	414	15
Orange	1 medium	311	2
Orange juice	1 cup	496	3
Peach	1 medium	202	1
Peanuts (plain)	2½ oz	740	2
Potato	1 medium	504	4
Prunes (dried)	8 large	940	11
Raisins	¼ medium	271	10
Spinach	½ cup	291	45
Squash (acorn)	½ baked	749	2
Sunflower seeds	3½ oz	920	30
Sweet potato	1 small	367	15
Tomato	1 small	244	3
Watermelon	1 slice (approx. 6½ in)	600	6

Adapted from *Health & Nutrition Newsletter*, vol. 1, no. 2 (February 1985)

Cholesterol

High blood cholesterol, like high blood pressure, increases the risk of a heart attack. In recent years the relationship between cholesterol and heart disease has gained tremendous media and public attention. In fact, patients now ask me more questions about cholesterol than any other health factor. I also encounter considerable confusion and misinformation regarding cholesterol—so much, in fact, that I have decided to devote a separate chapter (see Chapter 12) to this subject.

Fad Dietary "Cures"

A large proportion of the millions of dollars spent on improved remedies is spent on dietary nostrums—everything from herbal concoctions (many of which can be toxic) to megadose vitamins. Every now and then a new "wonder" dietary aid is introduced to treat high blood pressure, and inevitably patients come flocking to my office to ask whether they can use it instead of their regular medications. While many of these remedies are harmless, a patient can suffer greatly if they are used in place of legitimate treatments. The public should be wary of the nutrition expert who keeps touting his special formula vitamins and directs people to his favorite drug store. This may be good for his pocketbook but may not benefit or may even harm his audience.

For centuries garlic has been promoted as a treatment for almost every ailment known to humans. In recent years folk medicine "specialists" have hailed it as a treatment for high blood pressure and its complications. While there is some minimal evidence that very large amounts of garlic may lower blood pressure, the evidence is certainly not strong enough to warrant a recommendation. (At least one researcher has discovered that blood pressures will not go up in susceptible rats if they are fed lots of garlic; we await more information in humans.) Garlic in small amounts is a culinary delight, but when it is taken in large doses, the effect on breath and body odor is probably more pronounced than are its health benefits.

Unproved remedies promoted for high blood pressure or other forms of cardiovascular diseases include lecithin, ginseng, megadoses of vitamin E, and many other substances. In general, be suspicious of a claim that a food or food extract has unusual medicinal powers. Remember, anyone with a chronic illness that is not easily cured by treatment is a sitting duck for the purveyors of fads. Be especially wary of those who tell you that hypertension can be controlled in most cases by vitamins or special diets, and that most people don't need medication. This simply is not true.

Summing Up

- Although important, diet alone is not the most effective treatment of high blood pressure. Don't be misled into believing that diet is all that is needed in most cases.

- Cutting back on salt (reducing your intake in half) helps lower blood pressure and also can increase the effectiveness of medication in some people.

- Excess salt probably does not cause high blood pressure in people who are not genetically sensitive to it.

Low-Salt Cookbooks

American Heart Association. *Cooking Without Your Salt Shaker.* Available through local AHA chapters.

Brenner, Eleanor P. *Gourmet Cooking Without Salt.* Garden City: Doubleday, 1981.

Prince, Francine. *The Dieter's Gourmet Cookbook.* New York: Cornerstone Library, 1979.

Roth, June. *Salt-Free Cooking with Herbs and Spices.* Chicago: Contemporary Books, 1977.

U.S. Department of Agriculture. *The Sodium Content of Your Food.* Publication number 001-000-04179-7. This lists the sodium content of 789 food and food products and is available for $2.25 (make check or money order payable to Superintendent of Documents) from:

    Superintendent of Documents
    U.S. Government Printing Office
    Washington, D.C. 20402

• Weight control is an important preventive step in controlling high blood pressure and reducing the risk of diabetes, osteoarthritis, and other disorders.

• Common sense and moderation should be the key to any dietary program for the control of high blood pressure and heart disease.

6

THE ROLE OF EXERCISE

For some people, exercise may be helpful as part of a treatment program for lowering blood pressure. Exercise is good for you and makes you feel better. It should be something you enjoy and do at your leisure. But in our headlong drive to institutionalize or reduce almost everything we do to a precise routine, we have turned exercise or conditioning into a commodity to be packaged and sold.

Not long ago the president of a manufacturing company came to see me for a general checkup. He had just turned fifty, and as often happens after a significant birthday, he was taking stock of his life. "Doctor, it's time for me to get into shape. I need a complete work-up and an exercise test." Obviously this was a man who was used to giving rather than taking orders.

It turned out he had just joined a cardiovascular fitness program designed for executives. The brochure advised that "In 47 minutes a day we'll give you a healthier heart for the rest of your life." It took little imagination to figure out that the pitch was aimed at the affluent, hard-driving Type A executive who kept careful track of every minute. Before he could actually begin his daily computerized workouts, the program required a physician's okay, hence his visit to me.

During the course of our conversation and later examination I could find nothing wrong with the shape he was in. He had enjoyed good health all his life, and despite the fact that he thought he was leading a sedentary deskbound job, he actually was quite active. He belonged to a tennis club and played two or three times a week. On weekends he did a lot of walking, and he and his family skied fairly often.

His weight, cholesterol, and blood pressure were normal; he did not smoke or have any other cardiovascular risk factors or symptoms. "I don't think you need a stress test," I told him. "I can find no reason why you shouldn't participate in a conditioning program so long as it provides for a gradual buildup in endurance." I could sense he was not convinced. He produced an article by the director of a cardiovascular testing laboratory asserting that anyone over the age of forty should have an exercise stress test before starting a fitness program. "Look at this guy's credentials," he said. "Do you mean to tell me he doesn't know what he's talking about?"

I pointed out that the article's author was in the business of giving two hundred-fifty to three hundred dollar exercise stress tests, and it might just be that he wanted as many clients as possible. An exercise stress test is recommended for a *sedentary* person before embarking on a *vigorous* conditioning program if he or she has specific risk factors (i.e., a history of heart disease, high blood pressure, diabetes, or cigarette use). There is no reason however for a healthy person without definite risk factors or symptoms to undergo such testing unless he or she plans to become a marathon runner. The profit motive behind unnecessary testing was something this businessman could understand. It hadn't occurred to him that promoting exercise and all the frills that go with getting people in shape had become a multimillion-dollar growth industry.

TABLE 6:1
Calories Used in Exercise

ACTIVITY	CALORIES PER HALF HOUR
Moderate	*100–175*
Bicycling (5 mph)	105
(6 mph)	135
(8 mph)	165
Walking (1 mph)	68
(2 mph)	105
(3 mph)	135
Gardening	110
Canoeing (2½ mph)	115
Golf (using power cart)	100
Golf (pulling cart)	135
Bowling	135
Rowboating (2½ mph)	150
Swimming (¼ mph)	150
Badminton	175
Horseback riding (trotting)	175
Square dancing	175
Volleyball	175
Roller skating	175
Vigorous	*Over 175*
Table tennis	180
Bicycling (10 mph)	195
(11 mph)	225
(13 mph)	330
Walking (4 mph)	195
(5 mph)	220
Ice skating (10 mph)	200
Tennis	210
Water skiing	240
Hill climbing (100 ft per hour)	245
Jogging (5 mph)	265
Skiing (10 mph)	300
Squash and handball	300
Scull rowing (race)	420
Running (5 mph)	310
(8 mph)	360
(10 mph)	450

Adapted from the President's Council on Physical Fitness and Sports, Washington, D.C.

Exercise—Vigorous Versus Moderate

In this era of sweating equals longevity, anyone who claims that the benefits of vigorous aerobic exercise have been greatly exaggerated is akin to an heretic. Regular exercise is great for you, and properly done, it helps the heart work more efficiently. But the fact remains, there is no proof that regular *vigorous* exercises such as running or jogging to target heart rates extends life, significantly lowers blood pressure in the large majority of hypertensive individuals, or prevents heart disease. On the contrary, there is plenty of evidence that some of these exercises cause knee, ankle, and other orthopedic problems. Some may even be dangerous. Moderate exercise, on the other hand, may provide the benefits of exercise without the risks.

Exercise and Blood Pressure

As stressed earlier, *moderate* exercise in combination with a low-salt and, if appropriate, a reduced-calorie diet is an important first step in the treatment of mild to moderate high blood pressure. Studies have found that this approach alone is successful in reducing the blood pressure to normal levels in about 15 to 25 percent of patients with mildly elevated blood pressures. How much of the blood pressure-lowering is actually due to exercise is impossible to say. Some of the studies that claim dramatic decreases in blood pressure after specific exercise programs have been short-term or poorly controlled. Others have involved highly motivated patients who were willing to undergo vigorous programs that most of my patients and probably the majority of persons are unable or unwilling to follow for long periods of time.

TABLE 6:2
Calories Consumed in Some Normal Activities

ACTIVITY	CALORIES PER HALF HOUR
Sitting/conversing	40
Lawn mowing (power mower)	125
Lawn mowing (hand mower)	135
Cleaning windows	130
Mopping floors	130
Scrubbing floors	170
Vacuuming	130

As for longevity, recent studies do seem to support the contention that exercise (not necessarily running or jogging) may have a beneficial effect. For example, Dr. Ralph Paffenbarger and his colleagues at Stanford University School of Medicine as well as researchers at the Harvard University School of Public Health have gathered statistics on 16,936 Harvard alumni ages thirty-five to seventy-four. Of these, 1,413 died during the follow-up period from 1962 to 1978. In reviewing the life-styles of these alumni, the researchers found that men who were physically active (in terms of numbers of calories consumed by physical activity per week) had the lowest mortality rates. Their report stated: "With or without consideration of hypertension, cigarette smoking, extremes or gains in body weight, or early parental death, alumni mortality rates were significantly lower among the physically active." Although the study did not specifically measure cholesterol levels, other studies have demonstrated an increase in the "good" or protective HDL (high-density lipoprotein) cholesterol levels in people who exercise regularly. How much was life extended among the exercisers? According to the report, "By the age of eighty, the amount of additional life attributable to adequate exercise, as compared with sedentariness, was one to more than two years."

Significantly, men with histories of high blood pressure had death rates twice those of men whose pressures were normal. A family history of early death from heart attacks increased the mortality risk by 29 percent compared with alumni whose parents both lived to sixty-five years or beyond. Cigarette smoking also significantly increased mortality. Obviously the *total* life-style and family history are also important risk factors.

As for exercise, the researchers found that moderate amounts made a big difference. Men whose jobs required climbing several flights of stairs a day or who just walked from office to office during the course of a day fared better than those who were more sedentary. Add to this leisure-time walking, bicycling, tennis, golf, swimming, shooting baskets, bowling and other common activities, and it's not hard to burn up about *2,000 calories in physical activity* each week. That is the number that this study suggested would reduce the death rate in active men compared with men who were sedentary. The distinction may seem trivial, but my point is, *it's not necessary to take up jogging, to do aerobic dancing, or to join an exercise club unless you are a person who needs to follow and enjoys a structured plan.* Table 6:3 shows how you can burn up more than 2,000 calories a week without an organized exercise program.

Interestingly, men who were vigorous exercisers and used up 3,500 calories or more per week in exercise activities actually had higher mortality rates than the less active ones. We should remember however that Harvard alumni are hardly typical of the average American, but this study does provide some data about the benefits of staying active.

Remembers that you can increase your physical activity by simple modifications in your daily routine. For

TABLE 6:3
How to Burn Up an Extra 2,000 Calories a Week

According to the authors of the Harvard alumni exercise study, "Men whose weekly physical activity energy output totalled 2,000 or more calories per week had a 28 percent lower . . . death rate (from all causes) than less active men." Here's how to burn those 2,000 calories a week without strenuous sports or structured workouts.

SITUATION	ACTIVITY	CALORIES PER WEEK
On the job or at home	Climbing 2 flights of stairs daily	300
	Walking 1 to 2 miles a day on the job	750
Leisure walking	1 to 2 hours or 5 miles per week	350
Moderate sports, like golf, tennis, swimming	2 hours per week	750
	TOTAL	2,150

example, park your car or get off the bus or subway a few blocks away from your office, and walk the rest of the way. Or walk instead of drive to neighborhood destinations. Take a half hour walk at lunchtime. This not only provides exercise but is also a good way to unwind and return refreshed for an afternoon's work.

The late Dr. Paul Dudley White, an eminent Boston cardiologist and early advocate of moderate regular exercise to prevent heart disease, commented in a lecture in 1927 at the American Medical Association meeting on the treatment of heart disease other than by drugs that "walking is probably the best exercise because it is easy for anyone to accomplish and easy to grade from the slowest, shortest walks to the most rapid and longest." Again in 1960 in a lecture at the Federation of Women's Clubs, he concisely summarized the values of exercise. "Healthy exercise," he said, "is valuable not only for the maintenance of good physiologic function in the body which includes the circulation, digestion, and breathing, but also mental clarity and a feel of good health. It is probably the best antidote we know for nervous tension." Dr. White walked and cycled regularly until he died at eighty-five.

The Exercise Boom in Perspective

In our national enthusiasm to promote jogging, aerobic dancing, and commercial exercise programs, we have lost sight of one of the real benefits of exercise—namely, an enjoyable activity to help us relax and change gears. There is little doubt that on the whole we are more sedentary than our ancestors. At the turn of the century most people earned their livings through some sort of physical labor. They walked to school, the store, and other places that today we reach by car, subway, bus, or other means of transportation. Mowing the lawn, cleaning house, and other tasks of routine daily living required physical effort. There was no incentive or need to don jogging shoes and take to the open road for a bit of exercise. Only the very wealthy with staffs of servants could lead sedentary lives. Today most of us have relatively sedentary jobs, and our homes are filled with laborsaving devices. We are too busy just to take a walk.

Today's exercise boom began in the 1970's, when Dr. Kenneth Cooper, the late Jim Fixx, and a few other runners began to publish articles and books on the benefits of exercise. There was little scientific data to support their claims that vigorous exercise increased longevity. The studies which they did cite compared mortality rates of people whose jobs involved physical activity—London bus conductors who went up and down stairs all day collecting fares, dock workers, or postmen who walked their rounds—with sedentary counterparts—bus drivers and office workers, among others. In a review of these early studies, some glaring shortcomings are apparent. Were there other differences between the bus drivers and conductors that might explain differing mortality rates? For example, were the drivers more apt to be overweight or cigarette smokers? Were they less outgoing or more tense? And if exercise protected dock workers and bus conductors from heart attacks, how do we explain the high cardiovascular mortality rate among the physically active lumberjacks of western Finland? Obviously other factors like the high-fat intake of the Finns, are involved. None of these studies had compared persons who were joggers or runners with others but had merely pointed out, as the Harvard alumni study did, that an active life is probably better than a sedentary life. Of course, almost everyone agrees with this. It is the definition of "activity" or "exercise" and its benefits that must be more carefully outlined.

Half-truths and myths about the benefits of exercise abound. For example:

HALF-TRUTH: Regular vigorous exercise increases your life-span and prevents heart attacks.

FACT: Not even joggers or marathon runners are immortal. Witness the tragic death of Jim Fixx while running. We have become a nation intrigued by the jogging mystique. We are told that if you follow a specific regimen (often computerized on a weekly or daily basis at some of the more expensive exercise clubs) and accumulate *x* or *y* points a week, for getting your pulse rate to a target of 120–150 depending on your age, for thirty to forty-five minutes three or four times a week, you will be protecting yourself from heart disease. *Maybe*—but no proof exists that this kind of vigorous program is any better for you than a less strenuous one. One of my friends jogs for thirty to forty minutes four or five mornings a week. He gets a high when he runs, and after his workout, he's ready for a busy day's work. I remember how uptight he was before he took up running; today he's relaxed and even more productive. For him, running is great because he enjoys it, it makes him feel good, and he *is* improving his heart's ability to respond to sudden demands (we call this conditioning). But there is no evidence that he is prolonging his life. There is a great difference between conditioning or making the heart more efficient and *preventing* heart disease. Most of us can derive the same benefits from brisk daily walks or participating in a sport that we enjoy.

HALF-TRUTH: Exercise is the key to successful weight reduction.

FACT: Exercise may be important, but you have to cut down on calorie intake to lose weight. Exercise burns up some calories, but as you can see from tables 6:1 and 6:2 it takes a great deal of exercise to burn off those 200 to 350 calories from an ice cream cone, a slice of pie, or other high-calorie food. Walking for forty-five to sixty minutes at a brisk pace of three to four miles an hour will burn up an extra 200–300 calories a day, or 73,000 to 109,000 calories if you walk an hour a day for a year. This equals about twenty to thirty pounds of body fat. In actual life, however, few people are likely to walk this much at this pace. If you need to lose thirty or forty pounds, it will take quite a while to get there by exercise alone. In fact, it's practically impossible if your food intake stays the same. Regular exercise combined with a commonsense reduction in food intake, however, does work. *Weight loss,* however it is accomplished, *remains the most important nondrug method of lowering blood pressure.* Of course, many people with high blood pressure are not truly obese, but many of them could lose five to ten pounds, and even this might help.

HALF-TRUTH: Exercise strengthens the heart

FACT: Exercise does make muscles larger and stronger, and since the heart is mostly muscle, vigorous exercise over time will increase heart muscle size. During exercise more oxygen is needed by the working muscles; the heart is required to beat faster and pump out more blood. Thus its work load is increased. If we exercise regularly, our hearts become more efficient and our muscles learn to pull out oxygen from the blood more easily. For example, a well-conditioned athlete may be able to run a mile and his or her heart rate may increase only from 60 to say, 100 to 110 beats per minute. In contrast, a person who is not well conditioned may have a heart rate of 140 or more beats per minute after running or jogging only a few blocks. If, for some reason, a conditioned person must respond to an emergency or run to catch a train, his or her heart is able to pump out more blood during each beat without difficulty. A poorly conditioned person may not be able to do this. However, those of us who exercise only moderately are also probably conditioned enough to handle most situations that call for increased heart work.

Normal hearts can sustain an increased rate and

work load without difficulty, but if the coronary arteries are narrowed by fatty deposits, the heart muscle that is beating at a rapid rate may suffer from a lack of oxygen. This can result in chest pain, shortness of breath, irregular heartbeats, and so forth. A regular exercise program for persons with heart disease will help moderate the increase in heart rate and prevent trouble.

HALF-TRUTH: Shoveling snow, running to catch a train in the cold, or other such unaccustomed activities increase the risk of a *heart attack.*

FACT: While it is true that people may die suddenly while engaging in these activities, the cause of death is more likely to be a severe disturbance in the heart's rhythm (a condition called ventricular fibrillation) than a heart attack. This results when a portion of the muscle doesn't get enough blood. Regular exercise may protect us from this type of catastrophe because the heart becomes accustomed to strenuous activity and is not as likely to suffer from a deficit in oxygen when it is stressed by our shoveling snow or running for a bus. All the problems relating to heart strain are aggravated by high blood pressure. *Elevated blood pressure increases heart work and the amount of oxygen needed by heart muscle.* That is a major reason why it is important to have a normal blood pressure.

Designing an Exercise Program

Throughout this chapter I have stressed that normal daily activities may be expanded to provide adequate exercise. Still, many people feel the need for a structured, specific exercise program or routine. I would discourage you from following the lead of the patient described at the beginning of this chapter. The notion that you can rush off from the office, change clothes, go through a set routine (probably while taking your pulse every few minutes), shower, and get back to the office in time for an afternoon meeting is hardly a relaxing or enjoyable approach to exercise. Instead, it becomes just another Type A activity in a day filled with Type A time-oriented pursuits. There may well be some people who actually enjoy this regimen, but for most of us, I recommend a more leisurely approach to exercise.

For my patients regular walking is recommended as an ideal exercise. It does not require any special equipment; all you need are comfortable shoes and a place to walk. Twenty or thirty minutes of brisk walking three or four times a week can be worked into almost everyone's life. Unlike jogging, running, or skipping rope, walking does not put undue stress on the knees, ankles, and other weight-bearing joints. (Swimming is also an excellent exercise that is easy on joints.)

Skipping rope, aerobic dancing, jogging, and running are acceptable for people who enjoy these activities and do not have orthopedic problems contraindicating them. Even people with normal joints, however, may find that after a time they begin to experience problems with their knees, ankles, and backs.

A stationary bicycle, a rowing machine, a walking treadmill, or a cross-country skiing simulator—all are acceptable alternatives to outdoor exercise. Unfortunately, many people find that they are bored by this type of exercise and the machines are eventually relegated to a storage chest. If you do get one of them, it's not necessary to buy the most expensive model or machine that measures your heart rate; these are fine for an exercise laboratory but not really needed for home exercising. Running in place at your bedside every morning is also a good way to improve fitness.

A few minutes of simple stretching exercises both before and after a workout are important to keep you limber and to prevent unnecessary stresses and strains on muscles and ligaments.

Types of Exercise—Dynamic, or Isotonic (Motion), or Static, or Isometric

The major cardiovascular benefits are derived from aerobic exercises. Aerobic exercise is a fancy name for exercise that requires motion and oxygen. It is amusing to hear all the fuss about special *aerobic* dance classes and *aerobic* swimming classes—to mention two vogues of the moment. All exercises that involve movement of muscle groups are aerobic. These differ from isometric (static) exercises such as weight lifting or Nautilus machine workouts, which are good for increasing strength and muscle size. If you are someone who wants to look good at the beach, or a football player or wrestler who needs the strength for his sport activity, these exercises are a big help, but they're not nearly as good as dynamic or motion exercises for cardiovascular conditioning.

Isometric (pushing) exercises are not recommended and may be contraindicated for people with high blood pressure or heart disease. This type of exercise, during which muscles are tightened, tends to squeeze the small blood vessels (constrict them) and raise blood pressure considerably. The work of the heart is greatly increased. I have actually recorded pressures higher than 250/140 in a weight lifter when he pressed more than 150 pounds; other researchers have noted even higher pressures. This added pressure puts a tremendous burden on the heart. In contrast, dynamic (motion) exercise may raise systolic pressures, but diastolic pressures may be lowered because blood vessels in the large muscle groups are actually dilated during this type of exercise.

In designing your own exercise program, you must start gradually, and then, as your endurance improves, slowly increase the time you exercise. Avoid exercising to the point of fatigue. There is no added benefit from totally wearing yourself out. Stop exercising and rest if you experience chest pains, dizziness, shortness of breath, or other symptoms. If these occur, it's a good idea to see your doctor.

Summing Up

• Regular exercise alone is not effective as a treatment for high blood pressure *except in a few instances.* It should be used along with other treatments.

• People with high blood pressure should avoid exercises that involve pushing or tugging (isometric exercise) such as weight lifting. This raises blood pressure and increases heart work. If blood pressure is being treated and is controlled, any other exercise is fine.

• Regular moderate exercise is beneficial because it makes the heart work more efficiently. You also probably will look and feel better if you exercise regularly.

• Jogging, running, and other very vigorous activities probably produce no added benefits over walking or other moderate exercises that involve motion in terms of increasing longevity or preventing a heart attack.

• You can incorporate exercise into your daily routine without investing in expensive equipment or an exercise club membership.

• Healthy people who have been moderately active and who have no cardiovascular risk factors such as cigarette use, high blood pressure, diabetes, or evidence of coronary disease generally do not need exercise stress tests before embarking on exercise programs.

7

DRUGS TO LOWER BLOOD PRESSURE

As a physician I tend to be rather conservative when it comes to using such terms as "wonder drug" and "medical breakthrough." For the millions of Americans with high blood pressure, however, today's variety of highly effective antihypertensive medications may truly be wonder drugs. They represent one of this century's most important medical breakthroughs. In the preceding chapters I described a suggested approach to treating high blood pressure with diet, exercise, and other behavioral approaches. Although *some* people with mild to moderate hypertension *can* control their blood pressures with these nonpharmacological treatments, the majority still require some sort of medication to achieve and maintain normal readings.

When I began my medical career in the 1940s, there was not a wide selection of blood pressure-lowering medications, and understanding how even these few medications worked was quite limited. Today, however, there are dozens of different drugs, and physicians can practically always find a combination that will work to lower blood pressure. Even though new antihypertensive drugs are constantly being developed and introduced, many of the drugs that were introduced in the 1950s and 1960s are still among our most useful medications.

One of the first patients to be treated with a modern antihypertensive drug was a fifty-year-old man from

Blood Pressure-Lowering Drugs—How They Act

Diuretics work primarily by increasing salt excretion by the kidneys. Salt loss lowers the volume of blood and the blood pressure. Salt depletion in the blood vessel walls may help dilate them.

Angiotensin converting enzyme (A.C.E.) inhibitors act to prevent production of angiotensin, a hormone that constricts blood vessels.

Beta blockers probably reduce blood pressure by reducing the output of blood from the heart (or perhaps by blocking the production of angiotensin).

Calcium channel blockers prevent the entry of calcium into small blood vessels; blood vessels "relax" and blood pressure is lowered.

Vasodilators and alpha blockers act directly on blood vessel walls to prevent narrowing or to stimulate dilation.

Centrally acting drugs act on the brain centers and decrease nerve impulses to blood vessels; dilation results.

Peripherally acting drugs act by blocking the effect of adrenaline at the nerve endings. Dilation of blood vessels results.

Finally, there are drugs that have several actions—for example, a vasodilator plus an alpha or beta blocker.

Ohio. He came to the Cleveland Clinic with a blood pressure of 230/146 and a markedly enlarged heart. He was so weak and short of breath that he could no longer carry on his duties as an executive in a soft-drink manufacturing company. He had heard of the pioneering work of Dr. Irvine Page, revered today as one of the founders of modern antihypertensive therapy, and decided to give it a try. Dr. Page and his colleagues at the Cleveland Clinic had been studying the effects of hydralazine, a potent drug that relaxes the smooth muscles in arteries, thereby widening (dilating) them and lowering blood pressure. Since it was clear that this particular patient would soon die of heart failure unless drastic steps were taken to lower his blood pressure, Dr. Page decided to give him this experimental medication.

Hydralazine works very quickly, within minutes of being injected into the bloodstream. Over the next few hours Dr. Page and his fellow researchers carefully observed their patient and recorded a steady decline in his blood pressure. Over the next few weeks he was given hydralazine by mouth, and his blood pressure stabilized. By the time he left the Cleveland Clinic, his shortness of breath, edema, (swelling of the ankles) and other symptoms had improved. Although his heart was still enlarged, he was able to return to work. It was not long before hydralazine was approved for general use, ushering in the modern era of treating high blood pressure.

Before this time the major treatments for high blood pressure were mostly dietary. A few drugs were being tried, but many had highly toxic effects that limited their use. Dr. Edward Freis of Washington, D.C., another notable pioneer in hypertension treatment, experimented with very high doses of a drug used to treat malaria. It helped some people, but most could not tolerate the side effects. Dr. Page also tried a number of other approaches, including inducing a form of typhoid fever in patients with malignant hypertension. The rationale was that the resultant high fever would dilate blood vessels and reduce blood pressure. Today such approaches strike us as somewhat ludicrous, but only a few decades ago they represented the only hope for relatively young patients who faced certain death from rapidly progressive hypertension.

Although hydralazine represented an important

step forward in the treatment of hypertension, Dr. Page and many of us recognized that it was not an ideal drug. Our research group began using the drug in 1951 and noticed that it caused headaches and a rapid heartbeat. The latter raised serious questions about how safe it was to use in patients with coronary heart disease. In addition, a fair percentage of patients developed a tolerance to its effects; after a few days or weeks blood pressures rose again.

In the early 1950s a number of other drugs were studied for their ability to lower blood pressure, and two of them were added to the list of approved drugs. One of these was reserpine, a drug made from the root of an Indian plant called rauwolfia. This drug lowers blood pressure by inhibiting the action of the sympathetic nervous system. Interestingly, both hydralazine and reserpine are still used, but they are no longer first-choice antihypertensive agents. In combination with a diuretic, however, they are effective. In the 1950's we also tested drugs that blocked other parts of the nervous system, but most of these proved impractical or downright dangerous.

A major step forward in controlling high blood pressure took place between 1956 and 1958 with the introduction of the first thiazide diuretics, a class of medications that is still among the most useful in treating hypertension. There are many different brands of diuretics; commonly used ones include chlorthalidone and hydrocholorothiazide. They are marketed under a number of different brand names including Hygroton and HydroDIURIL. (See table 7:1.) In recent years they have received rather poor press, especially as new drugs have come along. In my thirty-eight years of treating hypertensive patients, however, I have found that diuretics, given alone or in combination with other agents, can control high blood pressure in most patients, even those with severe hypertension. In addition, diuretics are generally safe and free of important side effects.

Before discussing the specifics of various drug regimens, I would like to lay to rest several common misconceptions about antihypertensive medications. First, *I want to stress that the vast majority of people on antihypertensive medications can and do lead perfectly normal lives.* There is a widespread notion that these drugs invariably cause some kinds of side effects. While it is true that any drug, including such commonplace medications as aspirin, can cause annoying symptoms, the large majority of hypertensive patients tolerate their medications well. When problems do occur, they can usually (but not always) be solved by an adjustment of the dosage or a switch to a different drug or combination of drugs.

A major part of the decline in stroke deaths over the last two decades is a result of the improved treatment of high blood pressure—with drugs. In addition, many thousands of people who would have been doomed to increasing disability from heart and kidney disease or an early death only a few decades ago are now leading normal, productive lives.

In the early days of my medical practice I saw many patients who had been told by their doctors to quit their jobs and lead quiet lives in the hope that the avoidance of stress would keep their blood pressures from rising. One patient who stands out in my memory was a forty-two year-old executive of a major corporation. About a year before coming to me, he had checked into a medical center for a complete physical examination, a common practice before the institution of the simplified approach to diagnosis that doctors use today. The checkup found that he had moderately severe high blood pressures (170–180/105–110). The doctors at this center favored

FIGURE 2: Sites of Action of Blood Pressure–Lowering Drugs

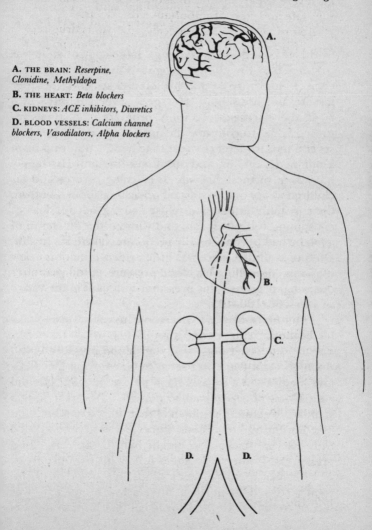

A. THE BRAIN: *Reserpine, Clonidine, Methyldopa*

B. THE HEART: *Beta blockers*

C. KIDNEYS: *ACE inhibitors, Diuretics*

D. BLOOD VESSELS: *Calcium channel blockers, Vasodilators, Alpha blockers*

a "naturalistic" approach and urged him to quit his job because "the stress was killing him" and to embark on a course of more relaxation, exercise, and special diets.

This particular man loved the fast-paced corporate world and was good at running a large company; he was frightened by the gloomy prognosis drawn by his physicians. Reluctantly he quit his job and set off to reorder his life and household. He spent several months in a rigid diet-exercise-relaxation program and then returned home to continue the new life-style. We saw him several months later. By that time he was suffering from a minor depression and absolute boredom. His family life was in turmoil, his wife threatening divorce and his children weary of the constant preaching about diet from their irritable father. He refused to eat out for fear of consuming too much salt, and without the diversion of a job he had become totally preoccupied with his health. On top of all this there was little evidence that his "new life" was controlling his blood pressure. A full year after the initial diagnosis, his pressures were still in the range of 155–160/100–105.

Our first task was to overcome his reluctance to take medication. "You've tried this other approach for nearly a year," I pointed out, "and your blood pressure is still too high. And you don't seem to be enjoying life. Let's give medication a try and see if we can get your life and your blood pressure back to normal." We prescribed a standard treatment regimen at that time: a combination of a diuretic and reserpine. Since he was so preoccupied with his health, we also taught him to take his blood pressure at home so he could follow his own progress.

Thanks to these medications, his blood pressure soon returned to normal. After a few months he was secure enough with the knowledge that his therapy was working that he returned to work. There have been several changes in his medications over the years, but even though he is again putting in long hours and leading a generally hectic life, his blood pressure has remained normal. He's a much nicer guy these days than when we first met him, and he's still active and healthy—thirty years after being sentenced to a life of boredom, early retirement and possibly early death. If you have high blood pressure, you don't have to be an invalid or an early retiree.

When and How to Treat High Blood Pressure

Physicians still disagree on when antihypertensive drug therapy should be started and what drugs should be used first. The 1988 recommendations from the National High Blood Pressure Education Program report stress that "the benefits of drug therapy outweigh any known risks to individuals with persistently elevated diastolic pressure above 94 mmHg, and to those with lesser elevations (90–94 mmHg) who are otherwise at high risk (e.g., men, smokers, patients with target organ damage, diabetes, hyperlipidemia [high blood cholesterol and other lipids], or other major risk factors for cardiovascular disease)." The report notes that "physicians who elect not to use drug therapy for patients in the 90–94 mmHg range should follow their patients closely. Some patients will progress to higher levels of diastolic pressure that clearly warrant antihypertensive drug therapy." In addition, the report states that some experts believe that drug therapy should be initiated in patients whose diastolic blood pressures remain above 90 mmHg.

I am one of many physicians who recommend drug therapy for any patient whose diastolic blood pressures

TABLE 7:1
Some Commonly Used Antihypertensive Drugs

TYPE OF DRUG Generic Name	STARTING DOSE AND SUGGESTED RANGE OF DAILY DOSE IN (mg/day)	
	Trade or Brand Name (Not all trade names listed)	*Starting—* *Maximum**
DIURETICS		
thiazides and related diuretics		
bendroflumethiazide	Naturetin	2.5—5.0
chlorothiazide	Diuril	125–250—500
chlorthalidone	Hygroton	12.5–25—50
hydrochlorothiazide	Esidrix, Hydrodiuril	12.5–25—50
indapamide	Lozol	2.5—5.0
methyclothiazide	Enduron	2.5—5.0
metolazone	Dialo, Mykrox, Zaroxolyn	2.5—5.0
Loop diuretics††		
bumetanide†	Bumex	0.5—2.5
ethacrynic acid†	Edecrin	25—50
furosemide†	Lasix	20–40—240
Potassium-sparing agents (usually used in combination with a thiazide)		
amiloride	Midamor	5—10
spironolactone	Aldactone	25—100
triamterene	Dyrenium	50—100

*The dosage range may differ from the recommended dosage in the package insert.
†This drug is usually given in divided doses twice daily.
††Larger doses of these diuretics may be required in patients with kidney failure.

TABLE 7:1
Some Commonly Used Antihypertensive Drugs

TYPE OF DRUG Generic Name	STARTING DOSE AND SUGGESTED RANGE OF DAILY DOSE IN (mg/day)	
	Trade or Brand Name (Not all trade names listed)	Starting— Maximum*
BETA-ADRENERGIC BLOCKERS		
acebutolol	Sectral	200—600
atenolol	Tenormin	25—100
betaxolol	Kerlone	10—20
metoprolol	Lopressor	50—150
nadolol	Corgard	40—160
pindolol†	Visken	10—40
propranolol†	Inderal	40—240
propranolol (long-acting)	Inderal LA	40—240
timolol†	Blocadren	20—60
ANGIOTENSIN CONVERTING ENZYME INHIBITORS (ACE INHIBITORS)†††		
captopril†	Capoten	25-50—150
enalapril	Vasotec	2.5-5—30
lisinopril	Prinivil, Zestril	5—30
CALCIUM CHANNEL BLOCKERS†††		
diltiazem*	Cardizem SR	60—240
nifedipine**	Procardia, Adalat	30—120
nifedipine	Procardia XL	30—120
nicardipine	Cardene	60—120
verapamil**	Isoptin, Calan	120—360
verapamil SR (long-acting)	Isoptin SR or Colon SR	120—360

*The dosage range may differ from the recommended dosage in the package insert.

†This drug is usually given in divided doses twice daily.

**This drug is usually given in divided doses two or three times daily.
Larger doses of these diuretics may be required in patients with kidney failure.

†††Several other Calcium blockers and ACE inhibitors may be approved for use within the next year.

TABLE 7:1
Some Commonly Used Antihypertensive Drugs

TYPE OF DRUG Generic Name	STARTING DOSE AND SUGGESTED RANGE OF DAILY DOSE IN (mg/day)	
	Trade or Brand Name (Not all trade names listed)	*Starting— Maximum**
VASODILATORS		
hydralazine†	Apresoline	50—200
minoxidil†	Loniten	2.5—50
pinacidil	Pindac	
CENTRALLY ACTING ALPHA BLOCKERS		
clonidine	Catapres	0.1—1.0
clonidine TTS (Patch)††	Catapres TTS	0.1—0.3
guanabenz†	Wytensin	4—24
suanfacine	Tenex	1—3
methyldopa†	Aldomet	250—1,500
ALPHA-ADRENERGIC BLOCKERS		
prazosin†	Minipress	1—15
terazosin	Hytrin	1—15
COMBINED ALPHA- AND BETA-ADRENERGIC BLOCKERS		
labetalol†	Trandate, Normodyne	200—1,200

*The dosage range may differ from the recommended dosage in the package insert.
†This drug is usually given in divided doses twice daily.
††This drug is administered as a skin patch once weekly.

TABLE 7:1
Some Commonly Used Antihypertensive Drugs

TYPE OF DRUG		STARTING DOSE AND SUGGESTED RANGE OF DAILY DOSE IN (mg/day)
Generic Name	Trade or Brand Name (Not all trade names listed)	Starting— Maximum*
PERIPHERAL-ACTING ADRENERGIC ANTAGONISTS		
guanadrel†	Hylorel	10—50
guanethidine	Ismelin	10—100
rauwolfia alkaloids (whole root)	Raudixin	50—100
reserpine	Serpasil	0.1—0.25

Adapted from the 1988 Joint National Committee Report on Detection, Evaluation, and Treatment of High Blood Pressure. Numerous other drugs are being studied. It is probable that several new ones will be approved for use in 1991.

*The dosage range may differ from the recommended dosage in the package insert.
†This drug is usually given in divided doses twice daily.

are consistently above 90 mmHg after a three- to six-month trial of diet and exercise. A number of extensive studies, including the Hypertension Detection and Follow-up Program Study, have shown that deaths from strokes and heart attacks can be reduced by lowering blood pressures that are consistently above this level. I also believe that when the systolic blood pressure is consistently higher than 140 mmHg, it should be lowered by medicines, if, of course, nondrug treatment hasn't worked.

The goal of therapy is to bring diastolic blood pressure to 90 mmHg or lower and systolic pressures below 140. Once it has been determined that antihypertensive medications are needed to achieve this goal, the next step is to design an appropriate treatment program. We now have a variety of drugs to choose from, and although there is some disagreement on which should be tried first, I believe that a simple treatment program can be established in almost all cases. Antihypertensives (blood pressure-lowering medications) fall into the following classes or categories:

Diuretics

These drugs, commonly referred to as water pills, work by increasing the excretion of sodium and water by the kidney. They thereby reduce the volume of blood in the arteries and veins and consequently lower blood pressure. Diuretics are classified according to their sites of action. The thiazides are the most commonly used and work primarily on the middle section of the network of tubes (tubules) that carry urine in the kidneys. The thiazides are well tolerated by most patients.

The more potent loop diuretics work on the part of the kidney called the loop of Henle, which is close to the area where waste products are filtered out. These agents usually are reserved for patients whose blood pressures are not controlled with thiazide diuretics or who have kidney complications or heart failure. A third class is called the potassium-sparing diuretics because they work on the part of the kidney tubules that is involved in the excretion of potassium. They are mostly used along with a thiazide or loop diuretic in order to help the body retain potassium while eliminating excessive sodium. (See Table 7.1.)

In recent years diuretics have been the object of adverse publicity, much of it generated by those who advocate the use of other drugs. In my experience many of the claims regarding adverse effects of diuretics are exaggerated. For example:

1. There have been suggestions that diuretics can have an adverse effect on kidney function. This may happen in a very small number of patients, but for the large majority, diuretic therapy results in *improved* or unchanged kidney function.

2. It has also been suggested that diuretics can have an adverse effect on cholesterol levels. While it is true that cholesterol levels may increase slightly and there may be a minor lowering of HDL—the so-called good or protective—cholesterol during the first few months of treatment, there is little evidence that these changes persist over a long period of time (more than a year) or that they lead to any adverse effects on longevity or heart disease.

3. There is some potassium loss following the use of diuretics in most patients, and in some, the decrease can cause symptoms of weakness or cramps. In most cases, this can be corrected by use of a combination of a diuretic and a potassium-sparing agent or by ingestion of potassium-rich foods or by potassium pills.

4. Other potential adverse effects such as impotence or reduced sexual desire (in both men and women) can be minimized *in most cases* by adjustment of dosages or the use of smaller doses of diuretics in combination with other drugs.

About 80 percent of patients, including those with moderately severe hypertension in the 160–170/105–110 range, will experience a definite reduction in blood pressure with diuretics used either alone or in combination with another drug. In addition to their high degree of effectiveness, other advantages of diuretics include their low cost and the fact that they are easy to use. Starting diuretic therapy is straightforward. As a rule only one or two doctor visits are necessary to arrive at the proper dosage. Most types of diuretics need to be taken only once a day, and some come in combination forms in which standard dosages of a diuretic and another medication are combined into a single pill.

Recently some experts have recommended special tests to determine which drug a patient should be started on. For the large majority of patients, this is not necessary. (See the accompanying box for specific suggestions as to when diuretics might be the preferred initial drug.) In short, I believe that a diuretic is a good first-step drug for most hypertensive patients. Some physicians will not use diuretics in patients with recurrent gout; these drugs tend to elevate uric acid in the blood, and this may precipitate or aggravate symptoms of gout. A few elderly patients become depleted of sodium and fluids after one or two doses of a diuretic. As with all drugs, these should be used in smaller doses in individuals over sixty years of age.

Beta Blockers

At present beta-blocking drugs are the second most widely used drugs to treat high blood pressure in this country. Propranolol (brand name Inderal) was the first beta blocker approved for general use in the United

Advantages of Diuretics

1. Lowers blood pressure when used alone in about 40 to 50 percent of cases

2. Effective in all types of patients—both blacks and whites as well as the elderly

3. Effective when used in combination with other drugs

4. Easy to take and relatively inexpensive

States. There are now six other beta blockers that have been approved for use and more will probably be approved within the next year or two. They all lower blood pressure in similar ways, but there are some differences among them.

When beta blockers were first introduced more than twenty years ago, they were used mostly to treat angina, the chest pains that occur when portions of the heart muscle do not get enough blood. Beta blockers work through our autonomic (automatic) nervous system, the system that regulates the heartbeat, breathing rate, and other involuntary functions. The name beta blockers comes from the fact that these medications inhibit or block the responses of certain nerve receptors (beta-receptors), which receive and act upon nerve impulses. For example, beta blockers prevent these receptors from signaling an increase in the heart rate during activity. Even when a person is resting, beta blockers slow the heart rate. In addition, less blood is pumped out with each beat. The use of beta blockers reduces the amount of oxygen required by the heart muscle and thereby enables someone with narrowed coronary arteries to be more active without getting chest pain.

The reduced amount of blood being pumped by the heart lowers blood pressure. Unfortunately, when the beta-receptors are blocked in the arm and leg blood vessels, these vessels may actually constrict and less blood gets to the fingers and toes. That's why some people who take beta blockers have cold hands and feet. In some instances, such as in diabetics or other patients who already have narrowed blood vessels in their extremities as a result of arteriosclerosis, the reduction in blood flow can produce symptoms of pain on walking. In these patients other drugs should be used.

In addition to possibly constricting peripheral blood vessels, the use of most of the beta blockers may cause constriction of the tiny muscles controlling the size of the bronchial tubes, which carry air to the lungs. This narrowing can result in symptoms of asthma in some allergic or "susceptible" patients. Several of the beta blockers, specifically pindolol (Visken), acebutolol (Sectral), and possibly atenolol (Tenormin) and metoprolol (Lopressor), may have less of an effect on leg and arm blood vessels and on the lungs than the other drugs in this group.

A beta blocker may be used alone as initial therapy for high blood pressure. Often, if a diuretic alone does not produce the desired fall in blood pressure, a beta blocker will be added to the regimen or substituted for the diuretic. About 80 to 85 percent of patients who are given a diuretic plus a beta blocker have their pressures lowered to normal.

Beta blockers seem to work best in younger patients with rapid heartbeats. Since beta blockers relieve the pain of angina, they may be preferred therapy for patients who have both high blood pressure and coronary artery disease. In general, blacks and the elderly do not respond as well to these drugs as they do to diuretics but there are exceptions. As noted, they should not be given to patients with bronchial asthma; they also may be contraindicated in people with blocked arteries in the legs.

Angiotensin Converting Enzyme Inhibitors

Usually referred to simply as ACE inhibitors, these are among the newest antihypertensive medications. They prevent the production of a powerful blood vessel constrictor, angiotensin II. Angiotensin is a chemical that plays a role in the control of blood pressure. Renin, which is excreted by the kidney in response to certain stimuli, helps convert angiotensin I (a relatively inactive substance) to angiotensin II, which causes constriction of blood vessels and stimulation of the hormone (aldosterone) that causes retention of salt and water. Blood pressure is raised by this combination of events (blood vessel constriction and retention of fluid). If the production of angiotensin II is blocked, blood pressure may be lowered.

The ACE inhibitors—captopril (Capoten), enalapril (Vasotec), and lisinopril (Prinivil and Zestril)—have received considerable publicity since they were introduced a few years ago. These drugs block the enzyme that helps produce the vasoconstrictor, angiotensin II. Many patients who have read about their effectiveness and low incidence of side effects request to be switched to these drugs. Though these drugs are effective and can be used as initial treatment in some patients, they, too, have side effects, such as rashes, a dry, hacking cough, palpitations, and headaches. They are also expensive, costing many times more than the diuretics or generic beta blockers, for example. There are some patients, such as those with hypertension and heart failure or diabetics with hypertension and kidney disease for whom they may be particularly appropriate. If, however, a person's blood pressure is well controlled with another drug without undue side effects, there is no reason to change to one of these newer agents simply *because* it is new. Black patients do not respond as readily to ACE inhibitors as white patients.

I have used the ACE inhibitors along with diuretics with good results, and *it is true that some patients feel better on these medications, compared with other drugs.* Also, sexual dysfunction may not be noted when they are used.

Calcium Channel Blockers

These are also new drugs. They lower blood pressure by blocking the entry of calcium into the blood vessel wall. Calcium is necessary for muscles to constrict. By blocking the passage of calcium into the muscle cells that control the size of arterioles, constriction is prevented and blood vessels relax and widen or dilate. The result is a lowering of blood pressure.

The calcium channel blockers available at present in this country are verapamil (Calan and Isoptin), nifedipine (Procardia), and diltiazem (Cardizem). Numerous other calcium blockers will probably be introduced for use over the next few years. These drugs are effective as initial treatment in about 30 to 40 percent of patients, but they are no more effective (and perhaps even less so in some patient groups) than diuretics or beta blockers. They are expensive and may require several doctor visits to establish an effective dose. Their most commonly noted side effects are listed in Table 7:4. Like many other drugs, they are especially effective when added to a diuretic.

As with the ACE inhibitors, these drugs have generated considerable publicity in nonmedical publications. For example, both ACE inhibitors and calcium channel blockers are widely described in the popular media as preferable to other drugs because of the low incidence of impotence associated with their use. The implication is that most antihypertensive drugs cause frequent sexual problems. For most patients this is not true ("Question of Sexual Function," p. 174). I have had patients who have never experienced sexual problems from their antihypertensive medications request a switch to these new drugs "just in case." This is not a good reason to change to a medication that is more expensive and that may not work as well. If problems do occur, then a change should be considered, but the adage "If it isn't broken, don't fix it" applies to hypertension treatment. After all, if a program is working, why change?

There are no data available as yet about the long-term benefits of using calcium blockers or ACE inhibitors in the treatment of hypertension, but some studies suggest special benefits from the use of these drugs in heart failure and kidney disease in diabetics (the ACE inhibitors) or in the reduction of heart size when calcium blockers are used. Many other blood pressure-lowering drugs also produce these benefits, and it remains to be proved that these newer classes of drugs are superior to the older ones.

Vasodilators

Vasodilators are drugs that widen, or dilate, arteries. This allows blood to flow more easily through the arteries; pressure or resistance is lowered, and blood pressure is reduced. Hydralazine (Apresoline), is the oldest of the vasodilators and is still used. Other vasodilators include minoxidil (Loniten), which has gained considerable public attention as a possible remedy for baldness. These medicines are rarely used alone in treatment and are usually given along with a beta blocker or other nerve inhibitor and a diuretic. They are generally given twice a day, and determining the best dosage may require several physician visits.

Some of these drugs are fast-acting and, when given intravenously or by injection are very potent blood pressure-lowering agents. Some, such as sodium nitroprusside (Nipride), are used mostly to control severe hypertension or a hypertensive crisis.

Alpha-Blocking Agents

These drugs work through the autonomic nervous system by blocking the alpha-receptors (receptors on the blood vessel wall that, when stimulated, cause narrowing or constriction of vessels). When they are blocked, dilation of the arterioles results. Because of their effect on blood vessels, they often are included among the vasodilators. Prazosin (Minipress) is the most widely used drug in this category. Terazosin (Hytrin) has recently been introduced.

Since prazosin or terazosin can cause fainting, especially after the first dose or when the dosages are being increased, care must be taken when use of these drugs is begun. Patients starting on either agent should be careful to avoid standing up suddenly since an abrupt change in position can cause a fall in blood pressure (orthostatic hypotension) and result in dizziness or fainting. Alpha blockers also inhibit the action of norepinephrine, one of the adrenal hormones that raise blood pressure in response to fright or other stress. These drugs are particularly useful for patients whose high blood pressure is caused by excessive amounts of adrenaline, such as in pheochromocytoma, the rare type of tumor that produces too many of these hormones.

Alpha blockers are rarely used as initial treatment. I usually reserve them for patients who have not had their blood pressures adequately controlled with other agents. These drugs are particularly useful for individuals with persistently elevated diastolic blood pressures.

Peripheral Adrenergic Antagonists

These drugs work by blocking the release of norepinephrine from the sympathetic nerve endings in response to stress. The oldest drug in the category is reserpine, which is made from the roots of the rauwolfia plant of India. In fact, these drugs were used in some Eastern societies for years because of their calming, sedative effect. Patients taking reserpine and other drugs in this category may note mental lethargy, depression, and sleep disturbances, such as nightmares. These effects usually can be avoided or minimized by taking the drug in small dosages along with a diuretic. Reserpine should not be used by anyone who has suffered bouts of mental depression.

The use of reserpine has decreased over the years, but I still continue to give it to selected patients, never as initial therapy but in combination with a diuretic. About 70 to 80 percent of patients respond with normal blood pressures. An added advantage is that reserpine is inexpensive.

Centrally Acting Drugs

These drugs work by reducing the number of nerve impulses coming from the brain to the sympathetic nervous system. They may lower heart rate to some degree but do not have a major effect on the amount of blood pumped out by the heart. They lower blood pressure by dilating the peripheral arteries. Drugs in this category include methyldopa (Aldomet), clonidine (Catapres), and guanabenz (Wytensin).

I rarely, if ever, use centrally acting drugs as initial treatment. They are usually given along with a diuretic if it has failed to lower blood pressure. Occasionally I use them as third or even *fourth* drugs in patients whose blood pressures are difficult to control. They can cause drowsiness, feelings of fatigue, muscle weakness, dry mouth, constipation, and other annoying side effects. They also may require several physician visits to arrive at a proper dosage. An adhesive tape-like skin patch that can be applied once a week and that contains enough clonidine to lower blood pressure may produce fewer side effects in some patients. In my experience, however, this is not a preferred way to treat most hypertensive patients. Clonidone has also been used as an aid to smoking cessation or in detoxification programs for alcohol or drug abuse. The drug helps minimize withdrawal symptoms.

Combination Drugs

In addition to single drugs, various combinations of blood pressure-lowering medications are available. These can be used after an effective dosage has been achieved. For example, if blood pressure is well controlled after several months of treatment with eighty milligrams of propranolol (Inderal) plus twenty-five milligrams of a diuretic such as hydrocholorothiazide per day, the patient might appropriately be switched to a drug that provides a combination of these two drugs in a single pill. In this instance, the drug might be Inderide, which contains eighty milligrams of propranolol and twenty-five milligrams of hydrocholorothiazide. There are many combination pills available that contain other beta blockers, alpha blockers, and ACE inhibitors along with a diuretic. (Some of the commonly used ones are listed in Table 7:2.)

Almost all the combination medications available contain a diuretic because this drug increases the effectiveness of most other antihypertensive agents. If your doctor has prescribed a combination that is not listed in the table, this does not mean it is inappropriate. Instead, it may be that you are on a combination that has been determined to work well for you, even though it is not one of the more frequently prescribed agents or the dosages are different from those in the listed medications.

I have found that the use of combination drugs makes treatment easier for the patient, who has fewer pills to take yet receives the same beneficial effect achieved with separate drugs. Occasionally the cost can be reduced by the use of this method of treatment. However, patients are rarely started on combination therapy because if side effects occur, it would be difficult to determine which agent is responsible. Also, it's possible that one agent alone would be sufficient to lower blood pressure. An exception might be for patients whose blood pressures are severely elevated. In these instances they might be started on a combination drug immediately rather than put through the process of trying one drug at a time.

TABLE 7:2
Some Examples of Combination Medications

BRAND NAME COMBINATION	CONTAINS THIS DIURETIC	PLUS THIS MEDICATION
Aldoril 15*	hydrochlorothiazide (15 mg)	methyldopa (250 mg)
Apresazide 25/25*	hydrochlorothiazide (25 mg)	hydralazine (25 mg)
Capozide 25/15*	hydrochlorothiazide (15 mg)	captopril (25 mg)
Combipres 0.1*	chlorthalidone (15 mg)	clonidine (0.1 mg)
Corzide 40/5*	bendroflumethiazide (5 mg.)	nadolol (40 mg)
Hydropres 25	hydrochlorothiazide (25 mg)	reserpine (0.125 mg)
Inderide 40/25*	hydrochlorothiazide (25 mg)	propranolol (40 mg)
Inderide LA 80/50*	hydrochlorothiazide (50 mg)	propranolol, long-acting (80 mg)
Minizide 2*	polythiazide (0.5 mg)	prazosin (2 mg)
Normozide 200/25*	hydrochlorothiazide (25 mg)	labetolol (200 mg)
Prinizide	hydrochlorothiazide (12.5 mg)	lisinopril (20 mg)
Regroton	chlorthalidone (50 mg)	reserpine (0.25 mg)
Salutensin	hydroflumethiazide (50 mg)	reserpine (0.125 mg)
Ser-Ap-Es	hydrochlorothiazide (25 mg)	reserpine (0.1 mg), hydralazine (25 mg)
Tenoretic 50 or 100*	chlorthalidone (25 mg)	atenolol (50 or 100 mg)

*Other combinations available.

TABLE 7:2 (*continued*)

BRAND NAME COMBINATION	CONTAINS THIS DIURETIC	PLUS THIS MEDICATION
Timolide*	hydrochlorothiazide (25 mg)	timolol (10 mg)
Trandate H.C.T.*	hydrochlorothiazide (25 mg)	lebatolol (100 mg)
Vaseretic	hydrochlorothiazide (25 mg)	enalapril (10 mg)

THESE CONTAIN A DIURETIC AND A POTASSIUM-SPARING COMPOUND

Aldactazide	hydrochlorothiazide (25 mg)	spironolactone (25 mg)
Dyazide	hydrochlorothiazide (25 mg)	triamterene (50 mg)
Maxzide	hydrochlorothiazide (50 mg)	triamterine (75 mg)
Moduretic	hydrochlorothiazide (50 mg)	amiloride (5 mg)

*Other combinations available.

Cost Considerations

While cost should not be the major determining factor in the choice of antihypertensive therapy, it must be a consideration. For the first time the data are beginning to show that increased cost has become a deterrent for a sizable number of patients to continue on a treatment program. If we are to lower blood pressure over a lifetime and prevent complications, it is necessary to avoid as many barriers as possible for the patient. Studies in Georgia and a recent Gallup poll have shown that almost 20 to 25 percent of patients are unable to refill their prescriptions as advised because of the costs. This may be due to the fact that more people are being put on the more costly medications. These newer drugs may be appropriate for patients who have been unable to tolerate previously used medications or those who have special problems. But for others there is probably no need to use them. Table 7:3 lists costs of commonly used antihypertensive medications, and estimates the approximate cost of drugs for a typical year of therapy.

Initiating Therapy

In the past few years there have been efforts to convince physicians to abandon the well-established step-care approach to treating hypertension. This is due in part, I believe, to the increased numbers and types of medications. Although the traditional approach may be modified for specific patients, on the whole, step care remains a logical and sound way to initiate and pursue treatment and to achieve good blood pressure control in a high percentage of patients.

Under this approach, in step one, a patient is started on a low dose of one of the following: a thiazide diuretic; a beta blocker; a calcium blocker; or an ACE inhibitor. If this does not produce the desired results, the dosage is increased. On the basis of long experience I still believe that a thiazide diuretic is most appropriate in about 70 to 75 percent of patients as initial (step one) treatment. In selected patients a beta blocker may be a better initial drug. I reserve the use of ACE inhibitors or calcium channel blockers for initial treatment or single-drug therapy in patients who have severe gout (which a diuretic may worsen) or those who have experienced

TABLE 7:3
*Approximate Cost of Some Antihypertensive Medications**

MEDICATION	AMOUNT (mg)	DOLLAR COST PER 100 TABLETS (BRAND NAME)**	APPROXIMATE DOLLAR COST PER MONTH***
DIURETIC			
Aldactazide	25	$25–30.00	$10–20.00
Hydroclorothiazide	25	3.50	1.00–1.50
(generic)	50	3.75	1.25
Zaroxolyn	2.5	30.00	10–15.00
Mykrox	0.5	32.00	10–15.00
Esidrix,	25	3.50	1.00–1.50
Hydrodiuril, etc.	50	3.75	1.25
Hygroton	25	7.50	2.50
	50	13.50	3–4.00
Lozol	2.5	50.00	15–20.00
Dyazide		35.00	10–12.00
Maxzide	—	45–60.00	15–20.00
Moduretic	—	35.00	10–12.00
COMBINATION DIURETIC AND OTHER ANTIHYPERTENSIVES			
Aldoril	2.50/25	32.00	20.00
Capozide	25/15	58–60.00	25–40.00
Combipress	0.1/15	25–45.00	15–25.00
Corzide	40/5	50–55.00	18–40.00
Inderide	40/25	30.00	10–20.00
Inderide LA	80/50	50–55.00	15–20.00
Minizide	2/0.5	30–35.00	20–30.00
Prinizide	12.5/25	110	35–70.00
Ser-Ap-Es	0.1/25/15	25.00	8–25.00

*Varies greatly among geographic area and pharmacies.
**Many brands have less expensive generic equivalents.
***Cost varies according to prescribed dosage.

TABLE 7:3 *(continued)*

MEDICATION	AMOUNT (mg)	DOLLAR COST PER 100 TABLETS (BRAND NAME)**	APPROXIMATE DOLLAR COST PER MONTH***
DIURETIC			
Salutensin	.125/50	$40–60.00	$15–30.00
Tenoretic	50/25	45–50.00	20–30.00
Vaseretic	10/25	80—85.00	35–40.00
ALPHA-ANDRENERGIC BLOCKERS			
Minipress	2.0	29.00	25–40.00
	5.0	50–55.00	40–55.00
Hytrin	2.0	70.00	50–70.00
ACE INHIBITORS			
Capoten	25	30–35.00	45–55.00
Vasotec	5	70–90.00	55–90.00
Zestril, Prinivil	10	55–60.00	45–50.00
CENTRALLY-ACTING BLOCKERS			
Aldomet	250	20.00	10–20.00
Catapress	0.1	15–20.00	20–30.00
Wytensin	4	40–42.00	40–50.00
BETA-ADRENERGIC BLOCKERS			
Corgard	40	40–45.00	15–40.00
Inderal	40	20.00	15–25.00
Inderal LA	80	35–40.00	20.00
Kerlone	10/20	69–100.00	20–30.00
Lopressor	50	30–35.00	15–35.00
Tenormin	50	40–45.00	15–30.00
Visken	5.0	50–55.00	30–45.00
Sectral	200	55–65.00	40–50.00
Normodyne, Trandate	100	22–30.00	30–45.00

*Varies greatly among geographic area and pharmacies.
**Many brands have less expensive generic equivalents.
**Cost varies according to prescribed dosage.

TABLE 7:3 *(continued)*

MEDICATION	AMOUNT (mg)	DOLLAR COST PER 100 TABLETS (BRAND NAME)**	APPROXIMATE DOLLAR COST PER MONTH***
CALCIUM BLOCKERS			
Calan or	120	$45–50.00	$30–50.00
Isoptin	20		
Cardene	20	40–45.00	35–75.00
Cardizem	60	45–55.00	55–65.00
Procardia	10	30–40.00	50–60.00
VASODILATORS			
Apresoline	50	30–35.00	35–45.00
Loniten	10	65–75.00	45–75.00
Pinacidil	–	–	–

*Varies greatly among geographic area and pharmacies.
**Many brands have less expensive generic equivalents.
**Cost varies according to prescribed dosage.

adverse reactions to a diuretic. ACE inhibitors or calcium blockers also can be used instead of beta blockers in patients with asthma, in diabetic patients who use insulin, or in patients who have various kinds of artery diseases. ACE inhibitors are especially useful, along with a diuretic, in patients with heart failure, and calcium entry blockers, like beta blockers, may be preferred in patients with angina.

If the desired blood pressure goal is not achieved, we go on to step two, which entails the addition of a small dose of one of the other drugs if a diuretic has been used initially. For patients whose initial treatment involved the use of a beta blocker, an ACE inhibitor, or a calcium blocker, a low dose of a diuretic is added. Again, dosages can be increased if blood pressure is not adequately controlled. If a beta blocker-diuretic combination doesn't work, an ACE inhibitor or calcium channel blocker may be substituted for the beta blocker. Or if an ACE inhibitor-diuretic combination doesn't work, a beta blocker may be substituted.

Under step three, a vasodilator or an alpha blocker is usually added to the treatment regimen. If an ACE inhibitor or a calcium channel blocker has not been substituted in step two, one or the other may be tried at this time. *Fortunately more than 75–80 percent of patients respond to the first two steps of the program and do not require the use of three or more different drugs.*

Under step four, guanethidine (Ismelin) or another medication such as minoxidil (Loniten) may be added. It should be noted that extremely few patients require the use of four kinds of drugs. Each of the different classes of drugs affect the mechanisms causing high blood pressure in a different way. Combining them allows these mechanisms to be altered.

During the period that therapy is being evaluated, I usually ask patients to return to the office about four to six weeks after treatment begins, unless they have only slightly elevated pressures (140/90 to 150/95–100) to begin with and no evidence of heart enlargement. For these latter patients, eight to ten weeks might be a reasonable time to see whether or not treatment has worked. This procedure can be followed because most of our patients are started on a diuretic, making it easy to arrive at an effective dosage. Also, side effects at the initial low dose level are usually minimal. The same approach can be taken with patients started on a once-a-day beta blocker, a long-acting ACE inhibitor, or a calcium blocker. Shorter-acting drugs in these last two categories require more frequent examinations. Patients with more severe disease may be seen in one week, or several different drugs may be started right away without waiting to see if one is effective by itself.

If a patient's blood pressure is normal on this return visit, he or she is instructed to continue on the medication and return in two or three months. If the blood pressure goal has not been achieved, the dosage and medications will be adjusted, and the patient will again be asked to return in four to six weeks. Usually a proper regimen can be arrived at in two or three visits; thereafter the patient usually returns every four to six months depending upon circumstances. The infrequent visits keep the inconvenience of treatment to a minimum, especially since my office is similar to many others in that patients do end up waiting longer than they or I would like them to.

The Issue of Side Effects

Medications to lower blood pressure are like any other drugs; there is always a certain risk of adverse reactions or undesired side effects. However, the actual incidence of problems has, in my experience, been greatly exaggerated. Many patients come to me fully expecting that their lives will change once they go on medication. Most are pleasantly surprised to find that the medications are very well tolerated, and when problems do occur, they usually can be remedied by alteration of the dosage or a switching of drugs. In fact, this is a major advantage of having so many different medications available, even if the large number is sometimes confusing to both patients and physicians.

As you might expect, different classes of blood pressure medications have different potential side effects. In selecting a drug, I consider the possible side effects and

Situations Where Certain Drugs May Be Preferred

If you are over age sixty	Diuretics and calcium channel blockers generally are more effective than beta blockers. Avoid drugs causing depression (e.g., reserpine or some centrally acting drugs). Prazosin, terazosin, guanethidine, or guanadrel must be used with care; orthostatic hypotension may result from their use.
If you are young	A beta blocker may be particularly useful in young patients, but exercise performance may be decreased in some individuals.
If you are black	Diuretics and calcium channel blockers are effective. Beta blockers and ACE inhibitors are less effective unless used with a diuretic.
If you are pregnant	Methyldopa, hydralazine, and beta blockers appear to be safe and effective. Most obstetricians are reluctant to use diuretics.
If you have heart failure	Diuretics, ACE inhibitors, vasodilators, and alpha blockers have beneficial effects.
If you have kidney failure	Loop diuretics (furosemide or bumetanide), metolozone, and vasodilators (especially minoxidil) are particularly useful. Potassium-sparing diuretics and guanethidine should be used with caution.

If you have angina pectoris	Beta blockers or calcium channel blockers are especially useful alone or with a diuretic (with a potassium-sparing component). Avoid drugs that cause rapid heartbeat (vasodilators) unless given with a beta blocker.
If you have had a heart attack	Beta blockers are the drugs of choice. They protect against a second heart attack. If blood pressure is not controlled, add a diuretic–potassium-sparing combination.
If you have diabetes	ACE inhibitors may have specific beneficial effects on the kidneys. Use of diuretics or beta blockers may adversely effect blood glucose levels, but this is not common or important in most instances. Alpha blockers are usually well tolerated. Beta blockers may mask symptoms of insulin shock. Potassium-sparing diuretics should be used with caution if you have kidney disease.
If you have had a stroke or ministroke	Probably you should avoid (or use with great care) drugs that may cause a decrease in standing blood pressure (e.g., alpha blockers like prazosin or drugs like guanethidine).
If you have asthma or chronic lung disease (emphysema, etc.)	Calcium channel blockers may protect against asthma that comes on after exercise. ACE inhibitors and diuretics are okay. Avoid beta blockers.

If you have Raynaud's phenomenon (white fingers or toes in cold weather)	Nifedipine, methyldopa, reserpine, diuretics, prazosin, and guanethidine may be used, but *avoid beta blockers.*
If you experience episodes of severe rapid heart beats*	A beta blocker or verapamil may be the drugs of choice. If blood pressure is not controlled, add a diuretic and make certain blood potassium levels do not decrease.
If you have bradycardia (heart rate slower than fifty beats per minute)	Avoid beta blockers, verapamil, and diltiazem.
If you have elevated cholesterol levels	Check blood chemistries periodically if you are taking beta blockers or diuretics.
If you have gout	Diuretics may precipitate an acute attack in predisposed patients and in those with kidney failure.
If there is a history of depression	ACE inhibitors, diuretics, vasodilators, alpha blockers, and guanethidine do not worsen or precipitate depression. Reserpine should be avoided. Centrally acting drugs (like methyldopa and clonidine) and beta blockers may cause or exacerbate depression.
If there is sexual dysfunction	Vasodilators, alpha blockers, calcium channel blockers, and ACE inhibitors may not affect sexual function as much as other antihypertensive drugs do.

*Some blood pressure-lowering drugs are also useful in treating other diseases.

If you have osteoporosis (thinning of the bone)*	Diuretics (except loop diuretics) may help preserve bone structure.
If you have migraine or angina	Beta blockers and calcium blockers may be helpful.
If you have heart failure	ACE inhibitors may be especially effective.

*Some blood pressure-lowering drugs are also useful in treating other diseases.

try to tailor therapy accordingly. For example, an older person is more likely to be troubled by dizziness or fainting from orthostatic hypotension (lowered blood pressure in a standing position) than a younger person. Thus, I would avoid medications such as prazosin or terazosin that are more likely to cause this side effect in elderly patients.

Sometimes I run across an unusual side effect that is not generally associated with a medication. For example, a relative of mine had been placed on an ACE inhibitor (captopril) along with a thiazide diuretic, which brought his blood pressure down to 135/85. At about the same time he developed a dry, hacking cough. At first I attributed the cough to an allergy because it was hay fever season. But the cough persisted into the winter, and he finally consulted a physician while in Florida. Thus began several weeks of testing—repeated X rays, sputum cultures, and a CAT scan. None revealed any lung problems or other reasons for the coughing.

At about the same time I was seeing a patient who was having similar problems. He, too, was taking captopril. I asked when he had first noticed his coughing, and checking back in his records, I noted that it coincided with his starting the drug. I decided to substitute another drug for captopril, and sure enough, the cough disappeared. I suggested that my uncle point this out to his physician, and within a week of his stopping the captopril, his cough disappeared.

Unusual and persistent coughs had not been noticed during the initial testing of this drug. This occasionally happens; drugs are tested in about two to three thousand patients prior to their release for general use. Occasionally, after a drug has been approved, a new side effect will turn up when it is used by larger numbers of people and for longer periods of time. For example, some side effects occur in one out of every thirty or forty thousand people and could easily be missed in a test on only three thousand patients. Fortunately these side effects tend to be rather rare and usually not too severe.

Frequently a side effect may not manifest itself (or disappear) immediately when a medication is started (or stopped). Thus patients or physicians do not connect the use of a drug and the symptom. I remember a patient who was on a diuretic and reserpine. His blood pressure control had been excellent for two years, and he appeared to be functioning normally. One day, however, his wife called to tell me that her husband was sleeping more and, over the past few months, had lost his enthusiasm for his job and family. In addition, he had lost all interest in sex, telling his wife that he was just too tired and working too hard. Insomnia and bad dreams when he did sleep also were upsetting him. He had not mentioned any of this to me, but not uncommonly the patient may be the last to notice such changes. Or he may attribute them to other factors such as age or increased pressure at work. Sometimes it is hard to separate what is drug-related and what is a result of outside factors. Reports of such symptoms always warrant investigation. If they are due to a drug's side effects, doctors can make appropriate changes and help eliminate them.

In this particular case the patient was experiencing a depression, which probably came from the reserpine. A small dosage of a beta blocking agent was substituted for the reserpine and the symptoms cleared up within four to six weeks. Table 7:2 lists the most common side effects of the different blood pressure medications. *These are the most common side effects noted, but this does not mean that they occur frequently.* Actually they occur in only about 10 to 15 percent of patients taking the drugs listed.

One added caution: All of us are subject to the power of suggestion especially when it comes to symptoms. The medical student syndrome is a well-documented phenomenon in which third-year students suddenly develop a baffling array of symptoms, invariably related to whatever disease or diseases they are studying at the moment. In looking back on my own student days, I recall being convinced I had at least one or more serious diseases—all in the space of six to nine months. Similarly many patients will develop symptoms of an adverse drug reaction after studying a list of the possibilities. This has been demonstrated in medical studies comparing the effects of a placebo, an inert sugar pill, and a real medication. In one study, for example, 15 percent of the patients placed on the placebo developed headaches, compared with 18 percent on the real drug. No one in this study knew whether he was taking a placebo or the active medication. In such a case it would be wrong to report that 18 percent of the people taking the drug can expect to suffer headaches. Actually only 3 percent more patients in the drug group than the placebo group had headaches.

TABLE 7:4
Some Possible Side Effects or Reactions to Commonly Used Blood Pressure-Lowering Drugs

These may be experienced by *a small percentage of people taking one or more of these medications.*

GENERIC NAMES	TRADE NAMES (examples)	SOME POSSIBLE SIDE EFFECTS
Diuretics		
thiazide or thiazidelike drugs	HydroDIURIL Esidrix or Hygroton or Zaroxolyn or Diulo or MyKrox	Weakness, muscle cramps, joint pains (gout), sexual dysfunction
indapamide	Lozol	
Loop		
furosemide	Lasix	
bumetanide	Bumex	
ethacrinic acid	Edecrin	
Beta Blockers		
atenolol	Inderal	Insomnia,
acebutolol	Lopressor	nightmares, slow
betoxolol	Tenormin	pulse, weakness,
propranolol	Sectral	asthmatic attacks,
nadolol	Kerlone	cold hands and
metoprolol	Corgard	feet, dizziness,
timolol	Blocadren	sexual
pindolol	Visken	dysfunction—
labetolol*	Normodyne or Trandate	varies with drugs
ACE Inhibitors		
captopril	Capoten	Skin rash, loss of
enalapril	Vasotec	taste, weakness,
lisinopril	Prinivil or Zestril	*cough*, palpitations, headache

*Is also an alpha blocker.

TABLE 7:4 *(continued)*

GENERIC NAMES	TRADE NAMES (examples)	SOME POSSIBLE SIDE EFFECTS
Calcium Channel Blockers		
nicardipine cardene		Swelling of legs, dizziness, flushes
nifedipine	Aladat or Procardia	palpitations, headaches, flushes
diltiazem	Cardizem	(constipation with
verapamil	Calan or Isoptin	verapamil or diltiazem)
Miscellaneous		
rauwolfia drugs	Reserpine Raudixin	Stuffy nose, nightmares, *depression*
methyldopa	Aldomet	Drowsiness, fatigue, depression, impotence, fever
hydralazine	Apresoline	Headaches, rapid heartbeat, joint pains
minoxidil	Loniten	Headaches, rapid heartbeat, excessive hair growth, fluid retention
guanethidine guanadrel	Ismelin Hylorel	A form of impotence, dizziness, diarrhea
clonidine guanabenz	Catapres Wytensin	Dry mouth, drowsiness, fatigue
prazosin terazosin	Minipress Hytrin	Faintness after first few doses, palpitations

Various combinations of drugs are also available. Almost all of the above medications are available in combination with a diuretic (see Table 7:3) Dyazide, Moduretic, or Maxzide are diuretics that contain medication that *prevents* potassium loss.

Not all available drugs or all possible side effects are included in this list.

Questions of Sexual Function

A certain number of patients taking blood pressure medications may encounter problems in sexual functioning, but this is not as common as many patients believe. Unfortunately, when sexual problems occur, they often go unmentioned and unsolved. Many patients and physicians alike are reluctant or embarrassed to discuss them. I recall one patient in particular, an attractive fifty-year-old woman who had been started on a low-dose diuretic for mildly elevated high blood pressure. Everything seemed to be going fine, but while we were chatting during one of her regular checkups, she blurted out, "Why didn't you warn me about this medication?"

When I asked her what was bothering her, she described a marked decrease in sexual desire and responses, to the point where the once active and fulfilling sex life she had shared with her husband had deteriorated to almost nothing. Further discussion seemed to indicate that her problems were related directly to her medication, not to any family or job situation. I substituted another medication, and at her next checkup she reported that everything was back to normal. Until then I had not been aware of many instances of sexual dysfunction among women on blood pressure medications. Now I make it a point to discuss sexual function with patients of both sexes, and I have found that about 5 to 10 percent encounter some difficulties.

Some drugs are more likely to cause sexual dysfunction than others. Studies indicate that the beta blockers, centrally acting drugs, and diuretics are the most common offenders. In contrast, sexual problems are relatively uncommon with the ACE inhibitors, calcium channel blockers, and alpha blockers. Thus, if we encounter a problem, it usually can be resolved by simply lowering the dosage of the possible "offenders" using small doses of two different drugs or changing to one of the medications less likely to cause sexual dysfunction, without a loss of blood pressure control.

It should be noted that not all sexual problems are due to medications. Many people receiving antihypertensive medication are in their fifties and sixties, a time when potency and sexual desire may be waning. Certainly their sex lives are not over, but at this time in life there may be a decline in libido in both sexes and a decline in male potency. Business problems, family crises, and many other emotional factors also affect sexual function. Diabetes often leads to impotence, which may occur even before the disease has been diagnosed. Heavy alcohol use and a number of medications in addition to blood pressure drugs can cause sexual problems. Thus, when difficulties occur, a bit of detective work to determine their source is in order.

I recently saw a sixty-one-year-old patient who complained of impotence. He had been on antihypertensive medication for several years without problems. About a year ago he started having difficulty achieving an erection. He attributed this to his medication and asked to be given another drug. The change in treatment failed to help, and since his blood pressure had been well controlled for some time and he probably was in no danger from temporarily stopping treatment, I decided that he should stop all medication during an upcoming vacation and see what happened. (Many men who have sexual problems at other times find that they are fine when they get away from their usual routine for a few weeks.)

In this instance the strategy did not work. I concluded that the problem was not due to his medication and referred him to a urologist. Again, a complete work-up could find no organic cause for his impotence. It was discovered that he was able to achieve an erection during sleep, so there was hope that he could regain his sexual function. The couple was referred to a sex therapist and was able to work through a long-standing problem that had only recently surfaced. Their satisfactory sex life has been restored, and he is back on medication with a normal blood pressure.

Every situation is different, and what works for one patient may not help another. For example, one of my patients is a forty-nine-year-old black attorney who had severe high blood pressure that was difficult to control. His heart was enlarged, and he also had some reduction in kidney function. After trying a number of different combinations of drugs, we finally brought his blood pressure down to normal with a diuretic, reserpine, and guanethidine, one of the very potent peripheral-acting nerve inhibitors. In a relatively short time he became impotent.

Over the next few months we tried other combinations of drugs, including beta blockers and ACE inhibitors, but these did not reduce his blood pressure adequately. We finally arrived at a partial solution: Every other weekend he would stop taking the diuretic and guanethidine. When he is off these medications, he is able to achieve fairly normal sexual function without a significant rise in his blood pressure. This may not be a perfect solution, but it is one that he and his wife can live with. Not all situations work out this well, and in some instances sexual dysfunction cannot be remedied, no matter what drugs are used or when they are given. In these cases, if the hypertension untreated is severe, the patient may decide that normal blood pressure is more important than his or her sexual activity. However I have had a few patients who have just decided to take their chances with untreated high blood pressure and have stopped medication because of persistent impotence. Fortunately, such instances are uncommon.

Some patients for unknown reasons react poorly to almost all the different blood pressure-lowering drugs. They experience weakness, light-headedness, palpitations, cramps, shortness of breath, constipation, headaches, rashes, and other symptoms from drugs that are *not supposed* to cause these types of reactions. Finding some combination of medication that works for them becomes a real challenge. It is frustrating, for example, to have a patient complain of palpitations or strange heartbeats when one of the beta blockers is being given because these drugs *usually* reduce the heart rate and prevent palpitations. It may be that the patient is imagining these effects, but when in doubt, I always change the treatment or dosage. Responses to medications are not the same, and individual differences should be respected.

Summing Up

• Today's wide array of blood pressure-lowering medications enables doctors to control hypertension in the vast majority of patients.

• Most side effects can be minimized or eliminated by an adjustment of dosages or a change of medications.

• New drugs are not necessarily better than some of the less expensive older ones, but they give treatment options and in some situations improve treatment results.

• Whenever symptoms are noted, they should be discussed with your doctor, even if they are not obviously related to an antihypertensive medication.

Aspirin and Heart Disease

Aspirin may not cause or cure hypertension, but this simple household remedy and the subject of doctor jokes for years may play a role in preventing strokes and heart attacks. It is important, therefore, for anyone with high blood pressure, or anyone who may wish to delay the occurrence of heart disease, to know the latest findings about this old new miracle drug. Physicians in ancient times recognized that chewing the barks of certain types of willow trees could relieve aches and pains. What they did not know was that the barks contained acetylsalicylic acid, the basic ingredient in aspirin.

Physicians have now recognized that aspirin may be beneficial in preventing heart attacks *and* strokes, and recent scientific studies seem to confirm this. Regular consumption of very low doses of aspirin—for example, a daily baby aspirin or even one-half aspirin every two days—alters the function of platelets (components of the blood that are an important element in clot formation) enough to help prevent some strokes and heart attacks. A recent study involving about twenty-two thousand healthy male physicians and coordinated by cardiologists at Harvard Medical School compared the heart attack rates among men who took low-dose aspirin with those of a matched group who took an inert substance (a placebo). Findings at the end of five years showed that doctors who took the aspirin had about 50 percent fewer heart attacks than the placebo control group. Given these dramatic results, the researchers decided to halt the study and give all the participants an opportunity to go on low-dose aspirin therapy.

More recent studies carried out by European researchers have found that small amounts of aspirin taken within a few hours after a heart attack and continued throughout the hospitalization and for one or two months thereafter seem to reduce mortality and the damage to heart muscle. These studies compared the use of aspirin alone and in combination with other drugs given to dissolve clots in the coronary arteries. In the groups of patients who received aspirin a lower mortality rate was noted.

Not all studies agree with these results, but the differences may result from the design of the research trial. For example, a study in Great Britain failed to demonstrate a decrease in heart attacks when aspirin was used. This study involved about five thousand physicians who took 500 mg (equivalent to about one and a half tablets) of aspirin each day, *more than twice the amount used in the American study*. Unlike small doses, large doses of aspirin may have little overall effect on preventing blood clots in the brain or heart. The British results may also lack the significance of the American trial because of the smaller number of participants.

The use of aspirin has been shown in many studies to delay or prevent further strokes in people who have had "minor" strokes or TIAs.

In view of these results, should everyone take *low-dose aspirin?* This would appear to be a logical recommendation, especially considering the high incidence of heart attacks in most industrialized countries. There are, however, some precautions to take. An individual with a history of an ulcer, frequent episodes of gastritis, or other stomach problems should be cautious about using aspirin on an ongoing basis. People with bleeding problems or who already are on blood-thinning drugs also should not take aspirin except under a physician's guidance. Likewise, *individuals with high blood pressure should be certain that their blood pressures are under control and at relatively normal levels before taking aspirin regularly.* Before you begin a regimen of aspirin, you should consult your doctor. There may be an increased risk of a brain hemorrhage if aspirin is taken regularly and blood pressure is high.

At present there are no data regarding the long-term benefits of aspirin use to prevent heart attacks in women. This might be because women are at lower risk of heart disease than men, and it would take a larger study over many years to demonstrate a difference in effect between aspirin and placebos.

8

BIOFEEDBACK, RELAXATION, AND OTHER NONDRUG THERAPIES

Not long ago a patient came to me with an article from a popular "natural" health magazine. The author was expounding on a familiar theme—namely, that Americans are overmedicated. As an example, the article cited the millions of Americans taking pills for high blood pressure when there is "ample evidence" that meditation and other nondrug treatments are just as effective and a lot safer than drugs. Typically the article failed to elaborate upon the "ample evidence" other than to quote some anecdotal accounts supplied by practitioners of alternative medicine and to misquote statements from various treatment studies.

In this era of New Age awareness, holistic medicine, and general nostalgia for the "good old days," a growing number of people are sincerely searching for alternatives to medication and other traditional therapies. This is particularly true for people with a chronic disease like high blood pressure, which can be controlled but usually requires lifelong treatment. If they could find an acceptable alternative, it might be better than taking medication. As noted in Chapter 5, salt restriction, exercise, and especially weight loss can produce a lowering of blood pressure in some people with mild hypertension, but the numbers of patients who benefit from meditation, biofeedback training, self-hypnosis, stress management, and other alternative nondrug treatments are not very great. Such approaches may temporarily lower blood pressure, but for most hypertensive patients, they simply are not effective in *maintaining* the lowered blood pressures.

In earlier times many hypertensive patients were given phenobarbital or some other mild barbiturate. Barbiturates are sedative-tranquilizers, and since it was believed that stress was a major factor in causing high blood pressure, there was a certain rationale to giving this type of medication. Of course, we now know that stress is not a major causative factor in the vast majority of cases and that tranquilizers and sedatives are of little benefit in lowering blood pressure over the long term.

Even if the barbiturates *had* been effective in lowering blood pressure, they needed to be taken several times a day, thus rendering their users walking zombies. In the days when there was nothing else available to lower pressures, patients might have accepted a little sleepiness in exchange for a strokeless future. Unfortunately sedation did not work in most cases.

Some of the newer tranquilizers, such as Valium or Librium, do not make people quite so sleepy, and they have been tried as treatments for hypertension, but with little long-term success. There are still some physicians who prescribe Valium or some other tranquilizer in the hope of lowering high blood pressure, but this is no longer accepted as effective treatment. Occasionally a tranquilizer or sedative may be needed to help a person through a particularly stressful or anxious period, but tranquilizers and sedatives should not be considered blood pressure-lowering drugs, nor should they be used on a long-term basis because of their habit-forming potentials. I have seen patients whose blood pressures were temporarily elevated as the result of a particularly stressful event and for whom tranquilizers were able to reverse the effects of stress (i.e., excessive production of adrenaline) and lower blood pressure. But these are situations quite different from chronic high blood pressure.

Hypnosis and Meditation

There is little question that hypnosis, meditation, or other relaxation techniques can temporarily lower blood pressure. During meditation, for example, respiratory and heart rates decrease and blood pressure drops. These techniques are useful in overcoming anxiety and stress and can also help break a cycle in which the body is pumping out too much adrenaline. A few minutes of meditation or brief self-hypnosis may help set a tranquil mood and improve a person's ability to concentrate, cope with stressful situations, or face a task with renewed energy.

Despite these recognized benefits, however, there is little evidence that relaxation techniques result in long-term blood pressure control. Studies have suggested that regular meditation or behavior modification using biofeedback training can lower mildly elevated blood pressures by about 5 to 6 mmHg. There are even a few studies that suggest there can be a greater lowering of blood pressure for as long as a year or more. Many of these studies, however, have not been well controlled, and we do not know if this can actually be applied to large numbers of patients.

Some of the behavioral modification techniques require considerable time and money to perfect. Biofeedback training is a good example. In this technique, electrical sensors and signals are used to teach a person how to control certain unconscious body functions. With a considerable amount of practice, people can learn to slow their heart rates, lower their blood pressures, and increase blood flow to certain parts of their bodies, among other things. Biofeedback requires a great commitment—the training is time-consuming, and the equipment is expensive—and the results are not always predictable. In my opinion, biofeedback training is most appropriate in very motivated patients with less severe hypertension who refuse to take medications or who have had serious adverse reactions to medications. It should not be used instead of drugs in patients with severe hypertension or in patients who have already developed complications, such as enlarged hearts or kidney damage, as a result of their high blood pressures.

Sometimes various relaxation techniques are useful adjuncts to traditional drug therapy. Some patients have been able to reduce their medication dosages by using techniques such as meditation and biofeedback training. Not only do they reduce their intake of medication, but they gain a more relaxed outlook and feel more in control of their lives. I have a number of patients who use the Benson relaxation technique one or more times a day to break the tension cycle. This involves sitting quietly with eyes closed and taking long, slow, deep breaths. At the end of each exhalation the person focuses on an image, a number, a face, or a place. Doing this ten to fifteen minutes at least once a day certainly can't hurt, it may make you feel better, and it *might* even make your pressure come down a little!

Fad Treatments

Every now and then a new health fad directed to hypertensive patients comes on the scene. A few years ago a company selling transcendental meditation (TM) as a definitive treatment for high blood pressure opened

Dr. Herbert Benson's Relaxation Response Technique

1. Sit quietly in a comfortable position.

2. Close your eyes.

3. Relax all your muscles, progressing from your feet to your face. Keep them relaxed.

4. Breathe through your nose. As you breathe out, say the word "one" silently to yourself.

5. Continue for ten to twenty minutes. You may open your eyes to check the time, but do not set an alarm. When you finish, sit quietly for several minutes, at first with your eyes closed. Do not stand for a few minutes.

6. Do not worry about achieving a deep level of relaxation. Maintain a passive attitude and permit relaxation to occur at its own pace. When distracting thoughts occur, don't dwell upon them, but return to repeating "one." With practice the response should come with little effort. Use the technique once or twice daily, but not within two hours after any meal, because the digestive processes seem to interfere with elicitation of the response.

To utilize this technique once or twice a day requires an ongoing commitment of time and effort.

Adapted from Herbert Benson, M.D., *The Relaxation Response* (New York: Times Books, 1984).

"clinics" around the country. The proprietors sent out advertising brochures calling TM an effective, proved treatment for high blood pressure. The courses were as costly as traditional therapy. The real danger, however, was that people would abandon the medical therapy that was controlling their blood pressures and adopt a treatment whose merits had not been scientifically proved.

"But, Doctor," one of my patients insisted, "it has been proved," and he showed me a brochure which claimed that TM's effectiveness against hypertension had been demonstrated in scientific studies. My colleagues and I failed to find references supporting this in the regular medical literature, so I asked the organization to supply its data. As suspected, there were no *real* data, at least, not of the kind we demand in scientific studies. Granted, the TM researchers could cite a certain number of patients whose blood pressures were lowered while undergoing TM training, but there was no long-term follow-up to determine whether the reduced blood pressures were sustained over time. Nor were there comparisons of TM with patients on a placebo relaxation program or other treatments. In fact, it was not certain that the modest reductions cited were actually due to the TM training. It is well known, for example, that after repeated blood pressure measurements over time *without any treatment,* lower readings are recorded in about 25 percent of people tested. These reductions can be attributed to many factors, including the simple fact that people become familiar with the blood pressure measuring devices and no longer feel anxious about having their pressures taken. By the way, this is a major reason that repeated blood pressure readings are taken before a diagnosis of hypertension is made or specific treatment suggested. Some of the miraculous results claimed for TM can probably be attributed to this phenomenon.

In general, relaxation techniques probably are most useful when combined with other therapies. To repeat, for the person with mildly elevated blood pressure—in the range of 140–155/90–95—there probably is no great danger in trying these techniques in lieu of drug therapy for a few months. But for people with more severe hypertension or with evidence of hypertension-related organ damage, these techniques should not be considered an alternative to traditional therapy.

Summing Up

• For *most* hypertensive patients meditation, biofeedback training, self-hypnosis, stress management, and other nondrug treatments are not effective in *maintaining* lowered blood pressures. These nondrug treatments, however, may temporarily lower blood pressure and in a few patients will produce good results over time.

• Tranquilizers should not be considered blood pressure-lowering drugs, nor should they be used on a long-term basis because of their habit-forming potential.

• Beware of fad treatments or treatments that promise a "cure" or good results in everyone. Most claims made by the companies promoting these treatments cannot be supported by scientific data.

9

WHAT IS YOUR ROLE IN TREATMENT?

Gone are the days when patients left the total responsibility for their medical care in the hands of their doctors. Today patients not only demand more say in their health care but also recognize that they bear some responsibility for their treatment. This is particularly true with a disease like hypertension, which usually requires lifelong management. In effect, the patient should be the doctor's informed partner, assuming responsibility for following his or her instructions and also being alert to signs of possible problems.

In many respects, successful management of high blood pressure is a team effort, with you, the patient, as the most important player. Your physician may be the captain, the one who calls the plays, but you're the one who carries the ball. Your spouse or partner, other family members, and, under certain circumstances, a pharmacist and perhaps a dietitian or other allied health professionals may become part of the team. No matter how many players on the team, you are the most important one because you are in charge of the day-to-day management of your high blood pressure regimen. Without your cooperation, treatment cannot be successful. Two recent patients illustrate this principle.

W. S., a forty-six-year-old truck driver, first learned he had high blood pressure when his dentist took a routine reading. He saw his doctor, who confirmed that his pressure was 180/110. He was put on medication, which brought his pressure down to a near-normal level of 125/85. At this point W. S. thought his hypertension was cured and he could stop taking the pills. Six months later he was admitted to a hospital with heart failure. He survived and is now doing fine. Had he followed instructions to keep taking his medication, and *if his doctor had been more diligent in making sure he did,* this patient could have saved himself a lot of trouble and worry.

In a somewhat similar situation, J. W., a fifty-three-year-old social worker, stopped her treatment on the advice of a well-meaning but uninformed friend. "Why do you keep taking so much medication?" the friend prodded. "You felt better before you started on all these pills." Under treatment, J. W.'s blood pressures had been 130/85; when she stopped her drugs without informing her doctor, her readings soared to 210–220/115–120. Within four months she had a stroke. She survived but remained partially paralyzed and probably could have escaped this fate had she stayed on her medication.

One of the most important steps you can take in managing your hypertension is to make sure that your doctor is one who believes that lowering high blood pressure really matters. This may sound obvious, but surprisingly, there are still a number of physicians who are not convinced that it's important to control elevated blood pressure. They persist in the old belief that a little high blood pressure is not necessarily bad and may even be beneficial as we get older.

As stressed earlier, we now have abundant scientific evidence proving just the opposite: That reducing even slightly elevated high blood pressures lengthens life and lessens the risk of such devastating complications as heart attacks, strokes, and kidney failures. Still, there are medical doubting Thomases who remain unconvinced.

A recent article in *The New York Times Magazine* (January 24, 1988) resurrected the ideas that: (1) higher than normal blood pressure may be helpful for some people in order to push enough oxygen to vital organs, (2) that specific treatment in mild to moderately severe hypertension may not be needed, and (3) therapy may actually be harmful. Whenever such an article appears, doctors' offices are besieged by patients who want to know whether they should stop their medication or why they were put on it in the first place. In such cases doctors should carefully explain why treatment is important and should be maintained. This, however, may be difficult if the physician is not personally convinced of the benefits of controlling high blood pressure.

So, first and foremost, make sure that your medical adviser is one who recognizes the importance of treating high blood pressure. If he or she tries to convince you that a little high blood pressure won't hurt, start looking for a doctor who is more up-to-date in the field of hypertension.

You must also make sure that there's a balance between under- and overtreatment. Just as some doctors neglect to treat high blood pressure adequately, so there are others who err in the opposite direction and overtreat it. In previous chapters I outlined an accepted approach to diagnosis and treatment: Unless your blood pressure is very high on the first visit, say, above 150–160/100 or you have other specific risk factors for heart disease, there is usually no need to start medication immediately. Instead, you should probably be told to restrict your salt intake, increase physical activity, and, if needed, stop smoking and begin to lose excess weight. You should return for a second checkup in about two or three months. Depending upon your blood pressure at that time, drug treatment may be started or you may be instructed to continue following the nondrug treatment for a few more months. Except in unusual circumstances, it is not necessary to undergo elaborate testing, twenty-four-hour monitoring, or other expensive procedures. Remember, you can say no if your physician wants to continue doing more and more tests.

Once your blood pressure is under good control, it will probably only be necessary to return for checkups about every four to six months. However, don't hesitate to ask your doctor questions during the interim periods. You should have a clear understanding of what you might expect from medication and be alert to possible side effects. As stressed in Chapter 7, the majority of people do not encounter serious or annoying adverse reactions or side effects, but occasionally they do occur. It is important that you contact your doctor if any unusual symptoms appear. In any event, *you should not stop taking the medication on your own, nor in most cases should you try to adjust your own dosage.* Under certain circumstances, however, there are exceptions. For example, severe symptoms may justify your stopping some types of medication and then contacting your doctor. Also, if you have been on a medication for some time, are monitoring your own blood pressure, and are well attuned to your body's reactions, you may be able to try a slight change in dosage. But I caution most patients to avoid too much self-doctoring. Also, some drugs, such as beta blockers or clonidine, should not be stopped abruptly, especially in people with heart disease, because sudden withdrawal may cause unusual heart rhythms, an increase in chest pain, or a marked rise in blood pressure.

You should let both your doctor and your pharmacist know what other medications you are taking before you start a new drug. This includes nonprescription allergy or cold pills, reducing aids, birth control pills, and high-dose vitamins and minerals. Many people have the mistaken notion that if a pill does not require a prescription, it's not really a medication. This is not true. Nonprescription cold and allergy pills or nosedrops, for example, can raise some people's blood pressures. Others may interfere with the action of your blood pressure medication.

Before leaving your doctor's office and your pharmacy, you should be absolutely clear about the instructions for taking your medication. It is best to have the instructions in writing. If you are to take a pill twice a day, find out if it should be before or after eating or if this matters. Also, ask what you should do if you forget to take one of your pills. Even the most highly motivated person can become so involved in an activity that he or she misses a dose. It's also a good idea to carry a spare prescription, especially if you are traveling. I've had many patients call me from out of town in a panic because they left their medications at home. Many times missing a dose or two is not critical, and nothing dramatic should be done to remedy the situation. Playing catch-up and taking extra pills the next day or two may, however, be dangerous.

At-Home Monitoring

Many patients ask me about taking their blood pressures at home. Generally, this is not necessary, especially if you have mild to moderate hypertension that is under good control. But some people are reassured if they know what their pressures are doing between physician visits. Some people insist on keeping daily graphs to chart the exact readings. This is acceptable, but there is a real risk of becoming obsessed with the numbers. After all, the emphasis should be on leading a normal life, not on constantly measuring your blood pressure. It is important to understand that now and then blood pressures can appear to be out of control. For example, they normally will rise during or immediately after periods of exercise and during periods of stress or emotional upset. They can also rise for a few days after you have eaten heavily salted foods or immediately after you have drunk a cup or two of coffee or chain-smoked several cigarettes. These rises tend to be temporary, and blood pressure will return to normal as the body "recovers" from the transient stimuli. Many patients who do at-home monitoring may become overly alarmed at changing or high readings and insist on seeing a doctor. By the time they get to the doctor's office, the pressures are likely to be normal once again. An occasional high reading at home is usually not a cause for alarm. Some at-home blood pressure machines are not as accurate as those used in the doctor's office and may give consistently high readings. If you do use an at-home machine, it's a good idea to take it with you once in a while when you go for a checkup so that it, too, can be checked. I've had several patients who have taken their pressures correctly and still had incorrect readings because they used poorly calibrated or overly sensitive electronic equipment.

We recommend at-home monitoring for patients whose blood pressures are difficult to control or who are experiencing symptoms such as dizziness that may be due to high *or* very low pressures. Sometimes it also is useful for a patient to do at-home monitoring when drug regimens are being changed or dosages adjusted. *Except in unusual circumstances, for example, if there are side effects or the hypertension is severe, weekly recordings are adequate to establish a trend. Once pressures have been brought under control, monthly readings are sufficient.*

How to Take Your Own Blood Pressure

If you do at-home monitoring, ask your doctor or nurse to show you how to take your own blood pressure using the kind of equipment you will have at home. You can then use the following step-by-step process as a refresher.

1. Make sure you have not consumed regular coffee or other sources of caffeine or smoked a cigarette for at least thirty minutes before taking your blood pressure. Both caffeine and nicotine can raise blood pressures (caffeine-free coffee is obviously not a problem).

2. Blood pressure may vary according to whether you are standing, sitting, or lying. Generally I recommend that patients take their blood pressure while sitting, although there may be some instances in which it should be taken immediately after standing, especially if you are experiencing dizziness or faint feelings when you stand up.

3. If you are sitting, rest your forearm flat on a table, with your sleeve rolled up. The upper arm, where you place the cuff, should be at about the same level as your heart (mid-chest level).

4. Wrap the deflated cuff around the arm about two to three inches above the bend in the arm (the junction of the upper arm and the forearm). The cuff should fit snugly around the arm.

5. If you are using a nonautomated machine, place the stethoscope in your ears, and place the diaphragm part of the stethoscope over the inside portion of the bend in your arm (the part of the arm nearest your body) at elbow level (it is now over your brachial artery). Remember, an automated machine has a stethoscope-like sensor and does not require a stethoscope. Begin to inflate the cuff. With the gauge in view continue to inflate the cuff to about twenty-five or thirty millimeters of mercury (or points) above your expected systolic pressure reading. For example, if your systolic pressure is usually about 130, inflate the cuff until the pressure gauge shows about 150–160. After you have inflated the cuff beyond your normal systolic pressure, you should no longer hear a tapping sound (blood being pumped through the arteries). In effect, the cuff is acting as a tourniquet to cut off blood flow through the artery; thus the lack of sound.

6. As you watch the pressure gauge, slowly let air out of the cuff. Listen carefully with the stethoscope for the first sound of a returning pulse. The pressure reading on the gauge at the point when you hear the first pulse sound is your systolic pressure. Make a mental note of this number, but keep listening through the stethoscope and let more air out of the cuff. When the pulse sound fades and disappears, the pressure on the gauge is the diastolic reading, or the pressure remaining in your blood vessels when the heart is resting. Remember there must always be some pressure in the arteries to keep blood flowing throughout the body. This procedure should take no more than twenty to thirty seconds. Keeping the cuff blown up too long or releasing the air too slowly may cause your fingers to become numb and tingly.

7. Wait a few minutes, and repeat the process to check that you get similar values. Numbers may differ by about 5 to 10 mmHg, but generally each reading will be fairly close to the other.

8. If you are using an automated device, follow the manufacturer's instructions. The principle is the same as outlined above, but you will not be listening for sounds through a stethoscope. Instead, you will note the numbers that appear on the electronic digital printout.

In some unusual circumstances out-of-the-office monitoring can be useful in the establishing of a diagnosis. A case in point involved a forty-five-year-old schoolteacher whose blood pressures were difficult to bring under control. When he was first diagnosed, his pressures were 155–160/95–100. During his checkups the readings ranged from 130/90 to 155/90. He complained of dizziness and periods of feeling faint at home. He was on a diuretic (HydroDIURIL), a beta blocker (atenolol), and an alpha blocker (prazosin). I was reluctant to increase his medication because I suspected his symptoms at home were caused by periods of low blood pressure.

He was instructed in how to take his pressures at home, and surprisingly, it turned out that his readings there were actually higher than they had been in my office. This is unusual, but it occasionally happens. With this information the medication dosage was increased, and his subsequent blood pressure readings both at home and in the office improved. His symptoms also were improved.

If you do at-home monitoring, you can use the same type of nonautomated equipment that most doctors use. These machines require that you use a stethoscope to listen for the proper sounds. Some people have difficulty managing both the cuff and the stethoscope. People who are hard-of-hearing may also have difficulty distinguishing the proper sounds. In such circumstances an automated device with a built-in stethoscope and a digital readout may be a better choice of equipment, even though some automated models may be less accurate.

Frequently Asked Questions

When you begin antihypertensive drug treatment, you undoubtedly will have many questions. You should not hesitate to pose these questions to your doctor, and if you do not understand the answers, ask him or her to explain them until you do. The following are some of the questions I hear most often from patients.

Q: How long will I have to undergo treatment?

A: There is no fixed answer to this, but for most patients some form of treatment is necessary for life. "Treatment" may of course just mean a diet, but for the majority of people, it means medication plus some behavioral changes. We often try to reduce the dosage of medication if normal blood pressures have been maintained for one to two years. In some patients pressures remain normal with about one half or one third of the original dosage. In others it is necessary to go back to the original dosage after a few months. Rarely can treatment be stopped completely and normal pressures be maintained.

In the 1960s my colleagues and I conducted a study to see what would happen if patients stopped therapy altogether. We took a hundred patients whose blood pressures had been under good control for more than two years and stopped their drug therapy. We did nothing else to alter their life-style patterns. Within a year ninety-six of the hundred were back on medication. Subsequent studies carried out in Chicago and Mississippi suggest that if patients are given nutritional and exercise guidance—for example, if they remain as thin as possible, reduce their sodium intakes, and increase their physical activities—as many as one half of the patients may be able to stay off drugs from one to three years. However, after that time most will be back on some medication. Psychologically this drug-free interval may be important for some people, but it also may be disappointing when they have to go back on specific treatment. Some patients may feel better when they are not taking medication, but most notice little or no difference. Thus, although short drug-free periods are possible, they usually cannot be sustained. If your blood pressures remain high enough during the period of evaluation to warrant drug treatment, it usually means that you'll be taking at least some medication for the rest of your life.

If a person is taken off medication, it is important that his or her blood pressure be checked periodically to make sure that it is still in the normal range. Sometimes blood pressures will bounce back rather quickly and may go even higher than before treatment was started. This is called rebound hypertension, and in certain circumstances it can lead to a serious hypertension problem. As noted, drugs like clonidine or guanabenz should not be stopped abruptly, because there is a possibility that a sudden rise in blood pressure may occur.

Q: How often will I have to see my doctor?

A: Once your blood pressure is under control, two or three visits a year should be sufficient.

Q: If I have high blood pressure, does this mean my children are going to develop it, too? Is there anything I can do to prevent that from happening?

A: As noted earlier, high blood pressure does tend to run in families, but there are commonsense preventive steps you can take to reduce the likelihood of your children's developing it. For example, watch their salt intake. Salt is an acquired taste. Infants and young children who are fed relatively low-salt diets grow up to be adults who don't heavily salt food or gravitate to foods that have a salty taste. A recent study in Philadelphia indicated that when young men and women aged eighteen to twenty-two with family histories of hypertension were placed on a high-sodium diet for just two weeks, their blood pressures rose to a greater degree than those who did not have such family histories. This finding tended to confirm that people with an inherited tendency to develop high blood pressure tend to be salt-sensitive. Maintaining normal weight, not smoking, and exercising regularly are other commonsense preventive health habits that you should try to instill in your children.

Summing Up

• Because hypertension requires lifelong management, patients must bear some of the responsibility for their treatment.

• Be sure that your doctor is one who believes in treating hypertension; even slightly elevated blood pressures can be a risk factor and should be controlled.

• Unless your blood pressure is very high at your initial visit to your doctor or you have other specific problems, there is usually no need to start medication immediately.

• If you are taking medication, you should not stop taking it on your own, nor in most cases should you try to adjust the dosage.

• If you do monitor your blood pressure at home, follow the proper guidelines for taking it and remember that electronic measurement devices may occasionally give falsely high readings. If you use an electronic blood pressure machine, take it with you once in a while when you go to the doctor's office. A comparison of the reading from your machine with that from an air or mercury column used by your doctor will tell you if your device is accurate.

10

WHAT ABOUT SMOKING?

No doubt about it, cigarette smoking is one of the leading causes of preventable deaths in the United States. By now virtually everyone is aware of the fact that smoking increases the risk of lung disease, chronic bronchitis, emphysema, and cancer. *But many people are still surprised to learn that cigarette smoking is also one of the three major risk factors for heart attacks and other forms of cardiovascular disease.* The surgeon general estimates that tobacco use is directly responsible for or a contributing factor in the deaths of about 345,000 people per year in the United States; 225,000 of these deaths are from heart attacks. This is more than twice the 102,000 smoking-related cancer deaths each year. If you're going to help yourself prevent heart disease by lowering your elevated blood pressure, you certainly must pay attention to this other crucial risk factor.

Despite repeated denials from the tobacco industry, there is a very convincing body of scientific data linking cigarette smoking and heart disease. In particular, the Framingham (Massachusetts) Heart Study has found that men who smoke have a tenfold increased incidence of sudden death from cardiac arrest compared to non-smokers. Smoking more than doubles the risk of death from heart attacks and strokes, and with high blood pressure, the risk is compounded.

Effects on the Cardiovascular System

Tobacco smoke contains about four thousand components. Nicotine is one of them. It is a powerful stimulant and the major addictive substance in tobacco. It is also one of the reasons why smoking is harmful to the heart and blood vessels. From the moment you take your first puff, nicotine enters the bloodstream via the lungs; its effects are noted fairly quickly. It takes only about ten seconds for nicotine to reach the brain, which signals the adrenal glands to pump out more epinephrine (adrenaline), one of the body's major stress hormones. This hormone causes the heart to beat faster and may raise blood pressure by narrowing the smaller, more elastic arteries. Thus there is less blood flow to the hands and feet. In some instances nicotine use may result in unusual heart rhythms or irregularities. This is why anyone with palpitations or skipped or extra heartbeats is told to stop smoking.

In the past physicians thought that most of these effects were temporary and that shortly after a person smoked one or two cigarettes, blood pressure and heart rates returned to normal. Today there is some evidence that long-term smoking may lead to more sustained rises in blood pressure, not only through its effects on blood vessels but also through its effects on certain adrenal hormones that control salt and water metabolism. Fluid may be retained, the volume of blood in the body may increase, and thus blood pressure tends to go up. Population studies have found that some smokers actually have increased levels of blood cholesterol compared to nonsmokers; this may contribute to their accelerated hardening of the arteries. Some researchers also believe that the body may form antigens against certain components of tobacco smoke and that this immune response may in some way injure the blood vessel walls and make them more susceptible to the buildup of fatty deposits. Finally, smoking may speed up the clotting mechanisms of the body, thereby increasing the risk of a stroke or heart attack.

It is probably not the tar or nicotine, however, that does the most damage to the circulatory system. Approximately one fourth of cigarette smoke is carbon monoxide, an odorless gas. When carbon monoxide is inhaled, it binds to hemoglobin in the red blood cells and significantly lowers the amount of oxygen that those cells can carry in the blood. This reduces the amount of oxygen available to various body tissues and, in particular, to the blood vessel walls. Remember, anything that damages the lining of the blood vessels or causes an irritation or inflammation within the vessel wall speeds up the deposit of fatty material beneath the vessel surface. In other words, it hastens the onset of arteriosclerosis, or hardening of the arteries, and thus the possibility of strokes and heart attacks. *A major culprit in damaging blood vessel walls is carbon monoxide. Regardless of what you smoke, it is the smoke itself that probably does the greatest amount of damage.*

"Safe" Cigarettes

Patients who smoke frequently ask me whether it will help to switch to a filtered cigarette or one that is low in tar and nicotine. Unfortunately the answer is mostly no. There is some evidence that a filtered brand or a cigarette that is low in tar and nicotine may reduce the cancer risk. But so far as the heart is concerned, there is no such thing as a safe cigarette. Even low-tar and low-nicotine brands produce harmful effects on the cardiovascular system. A person addicted to nicotine may simply smoke faster or more often and may smoke more of each cigarette in order to compensate for the lowered nicotine content in a particular brand. He or she may inhale more deeply, hence exposing the body to more carbon monoxide.

Some studies have found that filtered cigarettes may actually be *more* harmful to the heart and blood vessels than nonfiltered brands. The paper on filtered cigarettes is not as porous as that used in regular brands, and as a result, *more*, not less smoke may be inhaled. Studies have also found that smokers who use unventilated filters have lower levels of circulating oxygen in the blood than people who use regular cigarettes. This may explain why some population studies have found a higher death rate from heart attacks among smokers using unventilated filters than among those smoking unfiltered cigarettes. The next time you see an ad that suggests, "If you have to smoke, smoke a low-tar, low-nicotine, filtered cigarette," think twice. You may be misled into thinking that you're hurting yourself less by following the advice. Low-tar cigarettes may produce less irritation in the lungs, but not in the circulatory system.

Passive Smoking

The effects of passive smoking, or inhaling smoke from other people's cigarettes, are controversial, but it appears that passive smoking does have a harmful effect on people with heart disease. Recent studies by Dr. Scott Weiss and his associates at Harvard Medical School have found that side-stream smoke—the smoke from a cigarette, pipe, or cigar left smoldering in an ashtray—has a high level of carbon monoxide. Studies of passive smokers who inhale side-stream smoke show that they have reduced oxygen levels in their blood. The latest surgeon general's report on passive smoking estimates that it results in about five thousand preventable deaths each year. Although this is hard to verify, it is known that people who live with heavy smokers have an increased death rate from lung cancer and other smoking-related disorders. Consequently, when we treat our hypertensive patients who don't smoke, we try to convince them that their children and spouses shouldn't smoke either.

Pipes, Cigars, and Smokeless Tobacco

People who use pipes and cigars do not appear to have the same increased cardiovascular risk as cigarette smokers. This is probably due to the fact that they are not likely to inhale pipe or cigar smoke or to smoke as many hours of the day. It should be noted, however, that these tobacco products are not entirely benign: Pipe and cigar smokers have an increased risk of lip and mouth cancers. People who use snuff and other forms of smokeless tobacco expose themselves to large doses of nicotine and may become addicted to tobacco use. They also have an increased incidence of mouth and throat cancers as well as gum disease. However, smokeless tobacco probably does not have the same detrimental effect on the cardiovascular system as smoked tobacco, even though it may make the heart work harder and elevate blood pressure to a slight degree. The same is probably true of nicotine gum. Many smokers turn to nicotine gum as a substitute for cigarettes when they are trying to stop smoking. Instead of weaning themselves off the gum, some will continue to chew it for the nicotine effects. It is generally believed that this is not as harmful as smoked nicotine. In a recent study five out of a thousand persons using nicotine gum experienced palpitations, yet nicotine blood levels were not abnormally high in the gum users. People who have stopped smoking with the aid of nicotine gum should obviously try to stop the use of the gum, but in some cases the use of a few pieces of gum may be a lot better than going back to cigarettes.

Kicking the Habit

Many long-term smokers have the mistaken notion that the damage is done and stopping will do little good. *Nothing could be further from the truth. Even if you have smoked two or three packs a day for twenty or more years, you can reduce your risk of a heart attack—within two or three years after stopping—to a level close to that of someone who has never smoked.* You'll reap other benefits as well. I recently had a patient who came to me with a textbook of smoking-related problems. For more than twenty years this woman had smoked about two packs a day. Not only did she have high blood pressure and a high LDL (low-density lipoprotein) cholesterol, but she felt winded after walking just a few blocks. Although she was only forty-six years old, she was going through menopause, and another doctor had found evidence of considerable bone thinning (osteoporosis). (Women who smoke enter menopause an average of five years earlier and are probably more susceptible to osteoporosis than nonsmokers.) This woman also suffered from a chronic cough and repeated bouts of bronchitis. Almost as bothersome as her many medical problems was the accelerated wrinkling of her skin, another common problem among smokers. The wrinkling is caused mainly by the reduced surface circulation to the skin. However, in women the smoking-related reduction in estrogen and their early menopause also speed up skin aging. This particular woman had come to me because she was considering a face lift, and her surgeon had suggested that she get her blood pressure under control first.

For starters, I recommended that she stop smoking. "Oh, I've given up smoking dozens of times," she said, "but I've never been able to stick to it. And after all these years, what good would it do to stop now?"

I knew that other doctors had told her about the harmful effects of smoking to her heart and lungs, and she probably was bored by the repeated lectures. I repeated these dangers but then went on to emphasize what smoking might be doing to her skin and bone structure. She had not connected her premature aging to her cigarette use. I explained how smoking interferes with calcium and vitamin D metabolism and thereby may promote osteoporosis. I also explained how reducing circulation to the skin promotes premature wrinkling.

She obviously was interested in these "new" reasons to quit smoking, but she had one last argument, which I hear all the time. "I don't want to get fat," she said, "and everyone I know who quits ends up gaining weight."

People who stop smoking do tend to gain a few pounds. This may be due to an altered metabolism or to the fact that appetite improves and food tastes better when they're not smoking. Still, you can avoid weight gain by increasing exercise, eating low-calorie foods, and *going on a reduced calorie diet for one to two weeks before you attempt to stop smoking.*

Together we worked out a plan for her to stop smoking. She set a date to stop cold turkey in three weeks. She was going on vacation then and would be away from the pressures of her office. There would be other activities to divert her attention from the desire to smoke. She also knew she could count on the whole-hearted support of her husband and children, who had been urging her to stop smoking for years.

When I saw her three months later, she was pleased with herself. "I had a few jittery days," she said, "but nothing like I had expected." As a bonus, her hacking cough had disappeared, and she was walking farther without feeling short of breath. She had not gained weight, even though her appetite and enjoyment of food had improved. "I forgot just how good food tasted," she confessed. Still, she had managed to keep her weight down by eating smaller portions and increasing her exercise.

The increased exercise is also likely to help stem her bone loss and improve her skin tone. Obviously, stopping smoking is not going to erase wrinkles and recapture lost youth, but appearance certainly can be improved.

While concentrating on this woman's cigarette problem, we had also managed to reduce her blood pressure with the use of a small dose of a diuretic and a converting enzyme inhibitor. We had not specifically tried to do anything about her cholesterol levels, but her reduced food intake and increase in exercise also had lowered her LDL levels. This is a story with a happy ending, but many times we are not so successful: Patients are unable to stop smoking completely, and there is a weight gain despite efforts to control calories. The above situation, however, is an example of what can happen ideally.

Of course, the really important benefits of smoking cessation are not so apparent. Within a few months of a person's stopping smoking, the cardiovascular risk begins to decrease. For a person who smokes ten to twenty cigarettes a day for fifteen years, the risk of a heart attack can be reduced to that of a nonsmoker within six to nine months of stopping. Heavy smokers, two or more packs a day for twenty or more years, may require longer, but within two or three years the risk is almost that of a nonsmoker. All the damage to the lungs may not be repaired, but even here there is some improvement. Insurance companies have recognized that the risk of a heart attack or stroke is reduced in people who quit smoking and, as we all know, give policies with lower premiums to nonsmokers—even recent ones.

How to Stop

Since 1964 more than thirty-three million Americans have kicked the habit. Most, more than 75 percent, quit through their own efforts and without outside help. The remaining persons participated in some form of formal stop smoking program. Success, it should be noted, is not always achieved on the first attempt; relapse rates for smokers who try to quit on their own have been placed as high as 75 percent in some studies. Thanks to increased consciousness raising efforts, fewer people who quit resume smoking. The statistics for smokers who participate in formal programs are slightly better: Relapse rates range from 50 to 60 percent. However, the odds for permanent success improve with each successive attempt. The average smoker quits twice before permanently abstaining.

Quitting cold turkey—stopping all at once instead of cutting down gradually—seems to be the most effective and popular method of quitting smoking. The transition to a smoke-free life can be difficult, but with some thoughtful planning, going cold turkey can be accomplished. A positive attitude is the first step toward success. If you approach quitting as something you want to do and can do, your motivation will help get you through the initial difficulties.

It is important that you know *why* you want to quit smoking. Make a list that includes not only the well-known medical reasons but your own individual motivations, even the personal ones: You don't like the way your breath or your clothes smell, you don't want your kids to get the habit, and so forth. In addition, for several days keep a diary in which you record when and where you tend to smoke. For example, you may find that each morning you smoke two cigarettes during your coffee break. Understanding your smoking schedule will be of great help in your effort to stop. Another good prelude to quitting is to buy cigarettes one pack at a time. This makes smoking less convenient and maybe even more expensive.

Set a date for quitting which does not coincide with a time you will be under a great deal of stress. Vacation time may be a good choice. Whatever day you choose, though, stick to it. Support from friends and family can make this pivotal time even easier. Some smokers are hesitant to discuss their plans for stopping because they fear failure. However, most people, even nonsmokers, understand the difficulty of quitting smoking and will be supportive of your efforts.

As you plan psychologically to quit, you should also prepare physically. You can't smoke while you exercise, so begin an exercise regimen if possible. This does not have to be structured or organized; walks for twenty to thirty minutes a day may be all that is needed. Exercising routinely before you quit will also help control any post-quitting weight gain.

Now the hard part, actually quitting. You have thought about it, but now you must do it. The first few days after going cold turkey will, of course, be the most difficult. Nicotine withdrawal symptoms, such as headaches, irritability, an inability to concentrate, or cravings for cigarettes, can make quitting uncomfortable. Such symptoms last about one to two weeks, but the *worst* is usually over in the first three days. Although withdrawal symptoms are common, 40 to 50 percent of ex-smokers experience little or none of them. If you do have symptoms, ask your doctor about nicotine gum. In some cases a physician may actually prescribe the blood pressure-lowering drug called clonidine to minimize the problems of withdrawal. Recent reports suggest that a clonidine skin patch applied once a week for several weeks has been effective in reducing symptoms.

Some people, however, *never* get over the desire for a cigarette. Psychological cravings for cigarettes may last longer than any physical withdrawal symptoms, but over time they, too, will diminish. You can effectively distract your attention from cravings by seeking out places where smoking is prohibited, such as museums, theaters, or health clubs. Hiding all your ashtrays and throwing out any leftover cigarettes will also help. Many of these preparation and actual quit-smoking strategies are also valuable for smokers who choose to cut down gradually until they have quit completely or are participating in a formal program, such as SmokEnders. In these programs fewer cigarettes are smoked each day for about a week at a time until a specific date when all smoking is stopped. The gradual reduction in cigarette intake results in fewer nicotine withdrawal symptoms, but it also may be more difficult to accomplish.

According to a report by the American Cancer Society, about 30 percent of smokers who wish to quit believe they could benefit from some type of stop smoking program. Yet fewer than 30 percent of ex-smokers have actually participated in treatment programs, clinics, behavior modification therapy, or hypnosis.

One method which should be avoided by individuals with any cardiovascular disease is smoking adversion. This program forces a smoker to consume a number of cigarettes within a brief period of time. The underlying principle is that rapid and extensive smoking will make the smoker feel ill and thereby cause him or her to associate smoking with negative feelings. However, heart disease, asthma, and other medical conditions can be exacerbated by this kind of concentrated smoking. Individuals with any medical condition should consult their physicians before participating in any program which involves extreme changes in behavior or any type of drug. Programs which focus on health education and group support, however, pose no health risk. Nonprofit groups like the American Heart Association, American Cancer Society, and the Seventh-Day Adventist Church give out information and conduct stop-smoking clinics. SmokeEnders, Smoke Watchers, and other commercial programs boast a high rate of success, and the money you pay to enroll can be an extra incentive for success.

Summing Up

• Smoking more than doubles the risk of death from heart attacks and strokes, and if you have high blood pressure, that risk is compounded.

• Carbon monoxide, not tar or nicotine, causes the most damage to the circulatory system by promoting irritation and inflammation of the blood vessel walls.

• Despite the claims of companies producing filtered and low-tar and low-nicotine cigarettes, there is no such thing as a safe cigarette.

• People who use pipes, cigars, or smokeless tobacco do not appear to be at the same cardiovascular risk as cigarette smokers. However, pipe and cigar smokers do have an increased risk of lip and mouth cancers, and snuff users have more mouth cancer and gum disease.

• Quitting smoking can reduce your risk of a heart attack or stroke. Plan some stop-smoking strategies to help make the transition to a smoke-free life a bit easier, and consult your physician before beginning any stop smoking program which involves extreme changes in behavior.

11

WHAT ABOUT ALCOHOL?

About seven years ago a patient was referred to me because of uncontrolled high blood pressure. For the last two or three years his blood pressures had ranged from 150/100 to 190/120 mmHg, despite the fact that he was taking large doses of a diuretic and a beta blocker. His previous doctors could find no obvious reason for the poorly controlled blood pressure. At the time he was forty-six years old, relatively thin, physically active, and healthy-looking. His kidney function had been normal with no evidence of a narrowing of one of the arteries to a kidney, and there was no evidence of a hormone-secreting tumor or other organic cause for the continued high blood pressure.

In such cases I first try to determine whether the patient really is taking the prescribed medication. With this individual, however, there was no doubt that he was adhering to his regimen. During my physical examination the only abnormality I could find was an enlarged and soft liver. A doctor can detect this abnormality by feeling just below the ribs on the right side of the abdomen. The condition of his liver immediately raised a suspicion of heavy alcohol use. During our initial conversation he had said he had an occasional drink but had denied heavy drinking. More precise questioning revealed, however, that an "occasional drink" was actually three or four highballs every night, and instead of the usual one-ounce shot of whisky, each drink contained closer to two or three ounces.

These findings presented a definite clue to why this patient may have had "resistant" hypertension. Blood tests indicated early liver disease. The patient was not an alcoholic in the popular sense although he may well have been on his way to becoming one; he simply enjoyed having a few drinks to unwind before dinner each evening. He honestly was not aware that he was consuming more than five or six ounces of alcohol a day and that this might be the cause of his problem. Once he learned this, he had no difficulty in cutting his intake to about an ounce or at most two a day. This change in behavior was sufficient to resolve the blood pressure problem. The next time I saw him, his blood pressure was within the normal range. Within six months his liver function tests were back to normal, and two years later we were able to reduce his blood pressure medication by half. Today his blood pressures range from 120/80 to 140/90. As you might imagine, no doctor is successful in convincing all his heavy-drinking patients that they must cut down or they will continue to have a problem. Many drinkers are just not able to do this even with counseling, Alcoholics Anonymous, or other methods.

Alcohol per se is not considered a cause of hypertension, but heavy drinking seems to increase the risk of developing high blood pressure. Studies show, for example, that people who regularly consume five or more ounces of alcohol a day have a higher incidence of high blood pressure than nondrinkers. And as exemplified by this patient of mine, alcohol intake may make blood pressure control more difficult. It also may increase the risk of serious complications. Recent studies have found that people who consume the equivalent of five or more ounces of alcohol a day have an increased incidence of strokes.

How Much Is Too Much?

When I caution patients against heavy alcohol use, they invariably ask, "What do you mean by heavy?" Unfortunately there is no pat definition. Obviously a person who has five or six drinks a day is a heavy drinker by any definition. But there are a few people who can drink three or four ounces of alcohol a day and scarcely feel any effects, either emotional or physical. Their livers are able to metabolize this much alcohol without any *obvious* changes, and their mental abilities appear unhampered. They do not become decompensated alcoholics who are unable to hold a job, become overly aggressive or are unable to maintain personal relationships. More commonly, however, regular consumption of this much alcohol will eventually have an effect. Of course, there are people who are very sensitive to alcohol and will become quite drunk after consuming only an ounce or so. In short, alcohol tolerance varies considerably from person to person.

Over time even people who tolerate alcohol well will begin to show some effects of regular (daily) consumption of more than four or five drinks a day. Studies show that regular alcohol consumption in this range not only increases the risk of high blood pressure and heart disease but also damages other organ systems. Heavy alcohol consumption is a leading cause of liver disease. It also damages brain cells and can lead to a type of dementia similar to Alzheimer's disease.

Moderation is the key to alcohol use, as it is to most other things. There is no evidence that an ounce of alcool each day causes any harm to the vast majority of people. In fact, some studies indicate that a small amount of alcohol—for example, a glass of wine, a beer or two, or an ounce of whisky—may actually decrease the risk of coronary artery disease. This is probably due to the fact that small amounts of alcohol raise the protective HDL, or "good" cholesterol levels although we are not certain of the exact reason.

Unfortunately, when these studies were first announced, some overly zealous reporters misinterpreted the results as meaning that drinking can prevent a heart attack. Some wishful readers went even further and assumed that if a little is good, then more must be better. When it comes to alcohol, this certainly is not true. A small amount of alcohol may raise HDL cholesterol, but large amounts may have the opposite effect. Remember, too, that alcohol is high in calories: A gram of alcohol contains 7 calories, compared with 4 calories in a gram of carbohydrate or protein and 9 in a gram of fat. People who are trying to lose weight often concentrate on reducing the intake of solid foods, overlooking the calories in beverages of all kinds.

Alcohol can cause a rise in blood sugar. Thus people with diabetes—especially those taking insulin—should exercise special caution when drinking. This does not mean that diabetics can never take a drink, but they should understand how it affects blood sugar and must learn to adjust their food (and insulin) intake to "cover" the alcohol.

Alcohol Use by Hypertensives

Patients frequently ask whether they can have a drink or two if they are taking blood pressure medica-

TABLE 11:1
Alcohol and Calorie Content of Common Alcoholic Beverages*

Beverage	Calories	Alcohol (ounce
Beer, regular (12 oz, 4.5% alcohol by vol.)	145	0.46
Beer, light (12 oz, 4.5% alcohol by vol.)	100	0.39
Gin, rum, vodka, whiskey (1½ oz, 80 proof)	95	0.49
Gin, rum, vodka, whisky (1½ oz, 86 proof)	105	0.52
Gin, rum, vodka, whisky (1½ oz, 90 proof)	110	0.56
Bloody Mary (1 cocktail, 6 oz)	138	0.58
Gin and tonic (1 cocktail, 6 oz)	130	0.45
Martini (1 cocktail, 3 oz)	186	0.92
Screwdriver (1 cocktail, 6 oz)	150	0.42
Tom Collins (1 cocktail, 6 oz)	96	0.45
Whiskey sour (1 cocktail, 3 oz)	125	0.52
Wine, dessert (4 oz)	177	0.63
Wine, red (4 oz)	86	0.40
Wine, white (4 oz)	80	0.40

*The Joint National Committee on Detection, Evaluation, and Treatment of Hypertension defines moderate alcohol consumption as including a total of one ounce of alcohol daily—for example, about two beers, one martini, or two to three glasses of wine.

tion. The case cited at the beginning of this chapter illustrates how excessive alcohol intake can interfere with blood pressure control. There is no reason, however, why most well-controlled hypertensives cannot enjoy an occasional drink. Throughout this book we have stressed that the person whose blood pressure is under good control can lead a normal life. If a drink now and then is part of your regular routine, you probably can coninue in this pattern once your blood pressure is brought under control. Even if your pressure is not yet under control, a drink or two will probably do no harm.

However, you should be aware that alcohol and some blood pressure medications interact and the combination will increase certain side effects. Alcohol dilates blood vessels, especially in the abdominal area, hands, and feet. This is why many people feel flushed after a few drinks. When alcohol is mixed with certain blood pressure medications, this effect is accentuated. People taking beta or alpha blockers or converting enzyme inhibitors may complain of feeling dizzy or faint after taking a couple of drinks, especially if they are in a heated room or have had a heavy meal and then stand up suddenly. If you do feel light-headed or dizzy after a drink, you should sit down immediately and let the feeling pass. Drinking water will also help.

People taking some of the calcium channel-blocking drugs may experience palpitations or dizziness after drinking. These are not serious effects, but they can be annoying or worrisome if you don't realize what is causing them.

After an initial high, many people experience a mental letdown from alcohol. Alcohol is, after all, a depressant. This effect can be compounded if a patient is on blood pressure medications such as reserpine, methyldopa, clonidine, or guanabenz that work through the central nervous system. It's not unusual for patients on these drugs to become very down after a weekend of heavy drinking. A patient may blame the depression on the drug when in reality the alcohol may be equally or even more to blame.

The same is true of sexual function. Heavy alcohol intake *reduces* sexual capabilities. It may, as Shakespeare

advised us, increase the desire, but it also decreases th
performance. Men who drink heavily often experienc
impotence. If they also are taking blood pressure med
cation, especially one of those that may have the poter
tial to cause sexual problems, there is a tendency t
blame the drugs, not the alcohol. But when these me
stop drinking, they often find their sexual problems di
appear even though they are still taking the same bloo
pressure medication.

Another common problem among heavy drinkers i
that they may neglect to take their medication as pre
scribed. Poor blood pressure control results from suc
neglect. In such instances the patient and physician ma
blame the medication when, in fact, the real problem i
alcohol consumption and poor adherence to the trea
ment program.

On the whole most hypertensive patients learn t
listen to their bodies. If they feel dizzy after a drink o
two, they experiment with diluting the drink or sippin
it more slowly to avoid overloading the body with to
much alcohol. If a night of heavy drinking makes you fee
depressed for a week, your body is telling you to cu
back. Once you get to know how your body reacts to
combination of drinking and blood pressure medicatio
you can limit or adjust your alcohol intake accordingly
For most people total abstinence is unnecessary; insteac
moderation is the key.

The 1988 Joint National Committee on the Detec
tion, Evaluation, and Treatment of High Blood Pressur
notes that "excess alcohol intake may lead to elevate
blood pressure, poor adherence to antihypertensiv
therapy and occasionally to refractory hypertensio
Therefore, for controlling hypertension, those wh

drink should do so in moderation (no more than one ounce of ethanol daily; one ounce of ethanol is contained in two ounces of 100 proof whisky, approximately eight ounces of wine and twenty-four ounces of beer). Having served as a member of this committee, I agree with the statement, but if you are susceptible to alcohol or have any history or evidence of liver disease, abstinence is a must. If you have had a stroke or have a history suggesting low blood pressure when you stand up, you must also be very careful about alcohol intake.

Frequently Asked Questions

Q: Does alcohol raise blood pressure?

A: An intake of large amounts of alcohol produces dilation of blood vessels, which may actually tend to reduce blood pressure. But there is also an increase in heart rate, which tends to raise blood pressure and cancel the dilation effect. Consumption of large amounts of alcohol (more than 3 to 4 ounces of eighty proof whiskey per day) will result in a slight but significant elevation of blood pressure if ingested over a long period of time. This does not occur when alcohol intake is limited to less than 1 to 1½ ounces per day and does not occur in *all* heavy drinkers.

Q: If a person has heart disease, could drinking be dangerous?

A: Yes. In some instances an excessive amount of alcohol drunk over a short period of time, especially on an empty stomach, may produce unusual heart rhythms or a de-

crease in the ability of the heart to function properly, bu
most of the time a drink or two is fine.

Q: Should a person who has high blood pressure stop
drinking or drastically curtail consumption?

A: On the basis of current information, a patient with
high blood pressure *can* drink alcohol if he or she con
fines his or her drinking to less than approximately two
reasonably sized cocktails, eight ounces of wine, or two
cans of beer per day.

Q: Can alcohol cause cardiac arrhythmias?

A: Yes. Some people, after drinking just one drink, have
unusual or irregular heartbeats, probably caused by the
release of adrenalinelike substances. (These are not usu
ally serious but can be annoying.) Others, after one or
two drinks, will experience rapid heartbeats that may no
produce serious problems but might cause discomfort or
palpitations.

Q: Is alcohol consumption after exercise beneficial or
harmful?

A: There is no reason why a moderate amount of alcoho
(one to two beers or reasonably sized drinks) after exer
cise cannot be drunk by most people, other than those
with serious heart disease or those taking medications
that dilate blood vessels. (As noted, alcohol also dilates
the blood vessels.) In a patient with an abnormal heart
this intake of alcohol may cause a lowering of blood
pressure, faintness, and an increase in heart rate tha
could be dangerous. Fortunately this reaction is no
common. Alcohol in large amounts may enhance the
effect of drugs that a heart patient or a patient with high

blood pressure may be taking. For instance, a patient with high blood pressure who is taking a drug that dilates blood vessels may notice an increased effect if alcohol is consumed along with the drug—especially after exercise. Blood pressure may be lowered too much.

Q: Is there a connection between alcohol and strokes?

A: There is some information on this subject. Epidemiological studies, in which large numbers of people are observed over many years, indicate that excessive alcohol intake increases blood pressure and the occurrence of strokes. It seems appropriate, therefore, that alcohol should be limited to moderate amounts (fewer than two drinks of eighty-proof whiskey, eight ounces of wine, or two cans of beer daily) and that alcohol in large quantities should be avoided.

Q: How much alcohol consumption a day may be considered a safe amount for a normal person, for a hypertensive, and for a heart-disease patient?

A: I believe that the answer to all three questions is the same. The data listed above indicate reasonable and safe amounts. The intake of small daily amounts of alcohol may be protective against heart attacks and death from heart disease, but alcohol intake in large quantities over time may actually cause some heart muscle damage.

Summing Up

• Alcohol itself is not a cause of hypertension, but heavy drinking may increase the risk of developing high blood pressure.

- Alcohol intake may make high blood pressure more difficult to control. However, most well-controlled hypertensives can enjoy an occasional drink.

- Alcohol can interact with some blood pressure medications and result in side effects such as feeling flushed, dizziness, palpitations, impotence or feeling depressed.

12

THE CHOLESTEROL QUESTION

By now everyone is cholesterol-conscious, and indeed, there is little doubt that high levels of serum cholesterol (the amount that circulates in the blood) increase the risk of a heart attack. Since high blood pressure also increases the risk of vascular disease, it follows that people with hypertension should not only get their pressures treated but also strive for normal cholesterol levels. However, the definition of a "normal" cholesterol level is still open to debate—especially in those sixty years of age and older—and with all the recent publicity, encouraged by the National Cholesterol Education Program, I worry that this is just another area where needless anxiety may be produced and that too many people who have nothing to worry about will join the ranks of the worried well.

Despite all the media attention, the public as a whole is still confused over the meaning of cholesterol. For one thing, many people don't understand the difference between *dietary* cholesterol, which is what you eat, and *serum* cholesterol, which is what circulates in the bloodstream. Large amounts of dietary cholesterol may raise serum cholesterol in some people, but there are other factors that appear to be more important. These include genetics, obesity, gender, and the amount of calories and saturated fat in the diet. Cigarette smoking, excessive coffee consumption, stress, and the use of certain drugs also can affect blood cholesterol levels.

Many experts think that of all these, heredity may be the most important. Some of us can break all the rules and still have normal cholesterol levels. Others are born with genetic tendencies to produce too much cholesterol. Certain receptors in the liver play a major role in the elimination and manufacture of cholesterol. If you are fortunate enough to have effective receptors that will help get rid of extra cholesterol, you probably can eat all the eggs and red meat that you want and the amount of cholesterol in your blood will stay at low or normal levels. If you are less fortunate, it may seem that just looking at an egg raises your cholesterol levels. If your blood cholesterol is low (below 200) and you do eat lots of eggs and meat, you are probably one of the lucky ones with plenty of active liver receptors.

Actually about two thirds of blood cholesterol is manufactured by the liver, and only about one third comes from food sources. Men and women have about the same levels of total serum cholesterol, but men tend to have more of the "bad" LDL (low density lipoprotein) cholesterol, which is deposited along the artery lining, leading to atherosclerosis and increasing the risk of a heart attack. In contrast, women (especially before menopause) have higher levels of the protective ("good") HDL (high density lipoprotein) cholesterol, which may actually help cleanse the arteries of excess fatty material.

Obese individuals, especially men with potbellies (which describes many men over forty-five years of age), tend to have higher cholesterol levels than people of normal weight or than overweight women who are likely to accumulate fat in the buttocks and thighs. Abdominal fat is thought to be more active metabolically than fat elsewhere in the body (although some researchers discount this theory). We do not fully understand why potbellied men have high cholesterol levels.

In susceptible people, diets high in calories and saturated fats can raise blood cholesterol levels more than a diet high in cholesterol itself, a fact that many people find confusing. Saturated fats, the kind that are hard at room temperature, contain several specific acids that are not found in unsaturated fats. The unsaturated fats are liquid or soft at room temperature. These differences appear to account for the varying effects on cholesterol levels, although recent research indicates that one of these saturated fatty acids may not affect cholesterol as much as the others.

For years we have been warned to avoid eggs, red meats, and other rich sources of dietary cholesterol and been told that vegetable oils are better for us than lard, butter, or other animal fats. In general this is true, but newer studies highlight what some researchers have known for years: that foods made with some nonanimal fats, i.e. palm and coconut oils, which contain some of the most saturated fatty acids, can raise blood cholesterol more than butter or lard.

Many vegetable oils, such as corn oil or soybean oil, are made up of different kinds of fats (unsaturated) and have a less adverse effect on cholesterol than butter and lard, which are highly saturated. Olive oil and other mostly monounsaturated oils are safe to use in moderation if you are on a low-cholesterol diet (remember, they contain as many calories as any other fat). In short, it is impossible to make sweeping generalizations and say, "All vegetable oils are good," and, "All animal fats are bad." This simply is not true.

Many people mistakenly believe that fish, chicken, and other white meats have little or no cholesterol and that all red meats are automatically high in it. In reality, ounce for ounce, all these foods have almost the same amount of cholesterol. The difference lies in the

amounts and types of fat contained in them. Red meats
tend to have more saturated fat, ounce for ounce, than
fish or poultry. Also, the fat in fish and poultry is mainly
mono- or polyunsaturated and may have a beneficial effect on lowering cholesterol or improving the ratio of
HDL (good) cholesterol to LDL (bad) cholesterol."
Some researchers think that excess calories may be as
important as the types of fat in raising blood cholesterol.
(See Table 12:1 on Types of Fats in Common Foods.)

Food manufacturers have added to the general confusion over cholesterol. Suddenly "cholesterol-free" has
become a standard label on everything from margarine
and salad oils to peanut butter, cereals, and cookies.
Since these items do not contain animal products, the
only source of cholesterol, the labels are totally irrele-
vant. Still, labeling these foods "cholesterol-free" implies that they once had cholesterol, but now it has been
removed. It also implies that "cholesterol-free" foods
are in some way healthier than their counterparts that
are not so labeled. What the labels do not tell you is
whether or how much saturated fat, such as palm or
coconut oil, which can actually raise blood cholesterol
levels more, is in the product itself. A good example of
this is some of the "all-natural" breakfast foods that contain coconut oil.

In 1987 the National Cholesterol Education Program issued guidelines that defined "normal" and
"high" cholesterol levels and suggested specific treatment approaches. When blood is taken and cholesterol
levels are measured, the levels are reported as milligrams per deciliter (mg/dL); for example, a total cholesterol might be reported as 210 mg/dL or 280 mg/dL.
The average cholesterol level in American males is about
200–220 mg/dL. An earlier report had suggested that if
you are forty years of age or younger, a cholesterol level

TABLE 12:1
Types of Fat According to Saturation

TYPE	PERCENT POLYUN-SATURATED	PERCENT MONOUN-SATURATED	PERCENT SATURATED
Mostly Polyunsaturated			
Corn oil	59	24	13
Cottonseed oil	52	18	26
Safflower oil	75	12	6–11
Soybean oil	59	23	14
Sunflower oil	66	20	10
Mostly Monounsaturated			
Canola oil	32	62	6–11
Chicken fat	22	47	31
Lard	12	47	41
Margarine, hard†	29	35–66	17–25
Margarine, soft†	61	14–36	10–17
Margarine, tub†	46	22–48	15–23
Olive oil	9	72	14
Peanut oil	32	46	17
Sesame seed	40	40	18
Vegetable shortening, hydrogenated†	33	44–55	22–33
*Mostly Saturated**			
Beef fat*	11	4	52
Butter*	4	30	66
Coconut oil*	2	6	87
Palm oil/palm kernel*	2	10	80
Tallow*	5	44	51

Source: U.S. Department of Agriculture
*To be avoided.
†Varies according to manufacturer; check labeling.

above 240 mg/dL puts you at a high risk for heart disease; if you are over forty, a level of 260 mg/dL puts you at high risk. (See Table 12:2 for a recommended approach to managing high blood cholesterol. Table 12:3 lists common cholesterol-lowering drugs.) The more recent reports suggest that anyone, regardless of age, is at risk for early heart disease if levels are above 240 mg/dL.

I am a great believer in the fact that elevated cholesterol is an important risk factor for heart disease and that we all would be better off with low levels. All of us, regardless of how effectively our livers work, would remain healthier if we kept our intakes of fatty foods at a minimum. If high levels of cholesterol are present, we should certainly adjust our diets. The new report, however, ignores several facts when it defines cholesterol levels at which people are at "high risk." For example, it fails to note that an elevated cholesterol level in older people—those above sixty years of age—is probably *not* as great a risk factor as it is in younger people.

Cholesterol levels may vary a great deal—from day to day in the same person and from laboratory to laboratory. One or even two readings may not be accurate enough to classify you in a risk category. These facts should be kept in mind when you have your cholesterol levels checked. If it is above 260, make certain to have it checked again, and don't be overly concerned, especially if you are over sixty years of age. A second test may show levels 20 to 30 mg/dL lower. Even if blood cholesterol remains at a high level, you may not have to change your diet drastically or go on medication.

When it comes to cholesterol regulation, I urge my patients to follow the same kind of commonsense program recommended for weight loss or salt reduction. Cutting excess calories is an important first step in lowering blood cholesterol. Weight reduction will usually re-

TABLE 12:2
Suggested Approach to Managing High Blood Cholesterol

Note: A low-fat, low-cholesterol diet that does not provide excess calories will help prevent high cholesterol levels and makes sense for everyone.

Cholesterol Level	Recommended Action
Below 220–230 mg/dl.	You need not be concerned; recheck every one to two years. (Unless you smoke or have heart disease, hypertension, diabetes etc)
230–245 mg/dL	A specific low-fat, low-cholesterol diet is indicated. Cholesterol-lowering drugs probably are not indicated.
245–280 mg/dL	1. A specific low-fat, low-cholesterol diet that is also high in soluble fiber should be tried for four to six months. A low-calorie weight reduction diet should be initiated if person is overweight.
	2. If there is no change, check LDL and HDL levels. If LDL is above 190 mg/dL and/or HDL is below 45–50 mg/dL and person is under age sixty, cholesterol-lowering drugs may be considered, especially if there are other cardiovascular risk factors (cigarette use, diabetes, high blood pressure, and so on)
	3. If patient is age sixty or over, continue on diet alone, unless there are several other cardiovascular risk factors or heart disease, in which case medication may be initiated.

duce cholesterol levels. More specific restrictions of foods high in saturated fat and cholesterol also help lower blood cholesterol. It is not within the scope of this

TABLE 12:2 (*continued*)

Cholesterol Level	Recommended Action
280 mg/dL or above	1. A more rigid low-fat, low-cholesterol diet that is also high in soluble fiber is indicated for four to six months. LDL and HDL levels also should be checked. If LDL is above 190 mg/dL and diet is ineffective in lowering it to below 160 mg/dL, cholesterol-lowering drugs should be used, especially if other cardiovascular risk factors are present. The higher the level of cholesterol, the more important it is to treat it.
	2. If the person is sixty or older, medication still may be indicated, but in lower dosages and only after a good trial of diet and weight loss (if appropriate). A trial of small doses of omega-3 fatty acid capsules also may be indicated.

Note: Drug therapy is probably indicated in all persons under sixty years of age who have cholesterol levels above 300 mg/dL after three to six months of dietary treatment. These recommendations differ somewhat from those of the National Cholesterol Education Program—levels for concern, follow up and treatment that are listed here are higher than the program recommended. This in no way downplays the importance of cholesterol as a risk factor. It attempts to balance the proved benefits and risks of treatment.

Further information about the management of cholesterol can be obtained from local Heart Associations; the National Cholesterol Education Program; the National Heart, Lung, and Blood Institute C-200, Bethesda, Maryland 20892; and the Westchester Hypertension Foundation, 33 Davis Avenue, White Plains, New York 10605.

book to discuss the specific treatment of elevated cholesterol levels in detail, but Table 12:2 presents a brief overview of a suggested therapy plan.

Sometimes it is actually hard to convince patients they really need not be worried. Take, for example, the case of a very active seventy-eight-year-old retired schoolteacher. During a routine checkup I found that his total serum cholesterol was about 270, despite the fact that he had always been on a reasonably low-cholesterol diet. He had read that this put him in a high-risk category for a heart attack and asked me if he should go on cholesterol-lowering drugs. Since he had normal blood pressure and weight and was a nonsmoker with no signs of heart disease he definitely was not a candidate for drug treatment. Medication may not have been indicated even if he had had other heart disease risk factors.

I tried to reassure him that at his age a cholesterol level of 270 was not dangerously elevated and that the possible side effects from drug therapy were probably more of a risk than his cholesterol levels. What's more, he had a high level of HDL cholesterol (58 mg/dL), which further minimized his risk.

Still, he left my office worried. A week later I had a call from his wife. "He's driving me crazy," she said. "He found out I used one egg to make a batch of corn bread and practically accused me of trying to kill him!" Sadly a healthy, vigorous man was being unnecessarily transformed into an anxious, diet-conscious worrywart. I suggested that both he and his wife come in to discuss this "nonproblem," not because their diets were faulty but because they obviously needed reassurance. The session turned out to be important for the patient. He learned that a fraction of an egg in a piece of corn bread probably would have very little, if any, impact on his cholesterol. He also learned that the fiber in his favorite oatmeal cereal probably would offset the effects from an occasional slice of roast beef or a shrimp cocktail, two favorite foods he had all but eliminated from his diet.

The patient and his wife were given a booklet that listed the calorie, cholesterol, and fat contents of common foods and some general guidelines on how to plan meals with a balance of fats and cholesterol. The next time I saw my worried patient he seemed his old self. He was staying out of the kitchen and had simply continued his old habit of keeping his intake of butter, cheese, and fatty meats at a reasonable level.

Of course, if you do have a high serum cholesterol (above 250–260 mg/dL), you would do well to restrict your cholesterol and fat intake even more than you think you're doing (especially if you have other risk factors for heart disease—like high blood pressure). All of us are probably better off eating fewer prime ribs, hamburgers, marbled steaks, bacon, whole milk, butter, cheese, ice cream, and other foods high in saturated fats and calories. Unless your cholesterol is very high, however, there is no need for you to eliminate totally such foods from your diet. Instead, enjoy them in moderate amounts as an occasional treat, and make your dietary staples things like fish, chicken, veal, skim milk, margarine, low-fat cheese, pasta, vegetarian dishes, fresh salads, high-fiber cereals, vegetables, and fruits.

Part of the fallout of the present media campaign to lower cholesterol in everyone regardless of need is illustrated by a tale of woe related to me by a colleague. An eighty-three-year-old woman had seen him six months before, and her routine cholesterol level had been 295 mg/dL. Having just read the new guidelines, my conscientious colleague advised a low-cholesterol diet—no eggs, milk, butter, cheese, and so forth. The patient, who was a vigorous woman, lived alone on a fixed income and was used to having eggs, toast, and a glass of milk for dinner several times a week because these foods are inexpensive, easy to prepare, easily digested, and nutritious. When she tried to change her eating habits, she ran into problems: Fish was expensive, and she really didn't have the energy to prepare chicken dishes and other entrées. On her next visit she was quite upset, and her cholesterol levels were still 290. My colleague now suggested medication—nicotinic acid—in gradually increasing doses. Unable to take these pills because of dizziness, flushing, and headaches, the patient returned to the office a "nervous wreck." It was only then that her conscientious physician stepped back, considered what he had done, and told his relieved patient that perhaps it was okay to go back to her usual routine.

Actually that was not bad advice. Elevated cholesterol levels in older people may not warrant major lifestyle changes or the use of drugs. Until we have a simple and inexpensive way of lowering cholesterol, a major cardiovascular risk factor, I see no reason to upset the lives, or add to the medical expense, of our elderly citizens who have moderately elevated levels. I agreed with my colleague that he finally had done the right thing and that it just didn't make any sense to involve older individuals in the "cholesterol numbers game," certainly not at the levels of risk as defined by the National Cholesterol Education Program. In all treatment programs I attempt to balance the benefit of therapy against the risks. In most instances the benefits of treating a moderately elevated level of blood cholesterol in a person sixty-five or older have not been shown to outweigh the psychological, social, or medical risks of treatment. With hypertension, on the other hand, the benefits of treatment outweigh the risks at all ages.

Fiber and Cholesterol

Dietary fiber, or roughage, has long been advocated to relieve constipation and certain other gastrointestinal symptoms. Recent research also shows that some types of fiber may also help lower elevated blood cholesterol—specifically, the soluble or "sticky" fibers. Examples include psyllium, the fiber used in Metamucil and certain other fiber laxatives; pectin, which is used to thicken jams and jellies and is found in apples and some other fruits; oat and corn brans; and guar, a thickening agent used in ice cream and other processed foods.

Soluble fibers can lower blood cholesterol in two ways: First, they prevent the normal absorption of bile acids in the intestinal tract. These fibers bind or absorb the bile acids and remove them from the circulation to the liver. This action forces the liver to use up more of its own cholesterol in producing bile acids. Soluble fibers also can decrease cholesterol absorption; the liver must again utilize its own cholesterol stores to produce hormones as well as bile acids. Since more than two thirds of our blood cholesterol comes from the liver, these actions may lower blood cholesterol and may have a beneficial effect in preventing atherosclerosis, coronary disease, and heart attacks.

A recent study of twenty-eight middle-aged men suggested that if a low-cholesterol, low-fat diet does not reduce cholesterol to near-normal levels over a reasonable period of time, the use of soluble fiber substances might do the trick. When the men were given daily doses of Metamucil, the majority experienced a significant lowering of cholesterol. Scientists hope future trials will confirm this finding. The use of soluble fiber to lower cholesterol would be especially helpful to people who could also benefit from its laxative effects. This approach also is less expensive and entails fewer side effects than many of the cholesterol-lowering drugs. A word of caution, however: Too much fiber can cause bloating, intestinal gas, and discomfort. Start gradually; for example, a bowl of oatmeal or an oat-bran muffin for breakfast and an apple or two provide a good amount of soluble fiber.

It should also be noted that when it comes to lowering cholesterol, not all fibers are effective. When we say "fiber," most people think of things like bran cereals and other types of wheat or cellulose fiber. These may contain little or no soluble fibers and have little or no effect on cholesterol levels. Foods other than oat bran that are relatively high in soluble fiber include corn flakes, grape-nuts, bananas, corn, and beans. These foods may also contain insoluble fiber. Extra soluble fiber is not the panacea for lowering cholesterol levels that many people think it is, but it may help. More careful research on this subject is in progress.

"Cures"

In recent years, a number of special diets and treatments for high cholesterol have come on the market. One popular book, *The 8-Week Cholesterol Cure,* is promoted as being a sensible *nondrug,* dietary approach to lowering high cholesterol. The diet is a reasonable one, but since the book also recommends up to three thousand milligrams (3 grams) of nicotinic acid a day, a dose that many people find difficult to tolerate, the approach hardly can be described as "nondrug." Yes, nicotinic acid is a vitamin (as the book states), but more than a few of my patients have developed abnormalities in liver function and/or annoying side effects from it. I just do not believe that it is possible for most people to reduce cholesterol levels from above 240 to below 200 mg/dL and maintain them at these low levels by a diet and dosages of nicotinic acid that can be tolerated. I have been treating patients with high-fiber, low-fat, low-cholesterol diets plus nicotinic acid for many years and am not nearly as enthusiastic about the results of treatment as the author of *The 8-Week Cholesterol Cure.* This program will work beautifully in some patients and nicotinic acid is the first medication I and many physicians use if a diet proves ineffective after three to four months, but it is misleading to make it all seem so simple.

Fish-oil supplements are one of the newest of the dietary remedies. Oils from cold-water fish are high in omega-3 fatty acids. A few years ago researchers noted that Greenland Eskimos and certain fishermen who eat large amounts of fish enjoy a low incidence of hypertension, heart attacks, and other cardiovascular disorders, and they attributed this to the high amounts of omega-3 fatty acids in their diets. Early reports indicated that omega-3, indeed, may be beneficial in lowering cholesterol. It wasn't long before fish-oil supplements hit the market and with predictable results: Millions of these pills are now being sold, mostly to people taking them without medical supervision and before definitive proof that they really work.

More recent research shows that fish oil has only a slight effect on blood cholesterol levels. In fact, when taken in large doses, it may even have a detrimental effect. In large amounts fish oils may cause excessive thinning of the blood, increasing the risk of a bleeding. The American Heart Association warns against taking fish-oil supplements, especially in the suggested doses (ten to twelve capsules a day) of the products available. Some products contain large amounts of vitamin D, which may be toxic when consumed in excess. There have been some reports that omega-3 fatty acids may help lower blood pressure, but this has not been proved.

Population studies have found that people who eat fish two or three times a week have a lower incidence of heart attacks than those who do not. Many researchers believe, however, that any protective effect comes from eating the fish itself, rather than from just the oil. The American Heart Association recommends having two or three servings of fish a week as part of a balanced diet, an approach I endorse in most instances as making more sense than taking fish-oil supplements. I *have* advised the use of fish-oil capsules (the specific capsules like Promega that do not contain cholesterol) in small amounts—two to four capsules a day—in some of my patients with high cholesterol levels, especially if they don't like to eat fish. Occasionally I do see a decrease in the levels of fat in the blood in these patients. There is some research in animals to indicate that the use of fish oil may delay or reverse the process of hardening of the arteries. In small amounts this approach does *no harm.*

What should you expect as a result of dietary changes or the use of medication? If cholesterol levels are reduced to levels below 240—and they can be in many but not all people with the presently available therapies—you probably will reduce your risk of a heart attack. If you have already had one, you probably will reduce your chances of a second one. If your arteries already have fatty plaques (atherosclerosis), it is possible that some of the rust in the pipes will disappear. I say "probably" and "possible" because the scientific proof of this has not been clearly established except in certain groups of people, specifically middle-aged men who are high-risk. We have little data regarding the benefits of

TABLE 12:3
Most Commonly Used Cholesterol-Lowering Medications

Medication	Pros and Cons
nicotinic acid (Niacin, Nicobid)	Side effects (flushing, itching, liver problems) may limit its use. Takes several weeks to work up to effective dosage. Effective. Relatively inexpensive.
cholestyramine (Questran) or colestipol (Colestid)	Difficult to take; gastrointestional side effects may limit use.
lovastatin (Mevacor)	Easy to take. Very effective, Mild to moderate side effects. Expensive.
probucol, Lorelco, gemfibrozil (Lopid)	Probably not as effective in lowering total cholesterol and LDLs as other drugs.

lowering cholesterol levels in women or in persons over sixty years of age. We have far less data confirming the benefits of reducing fat levels in the blood than we do regarding the well-defined benefits of reducing elevated blood pressure. Until more proof is forthcoming (it may be within the next few years) and until we have easier to take and less expensive cholesterol-lowering medications, I believe that diet should remain the mainstay of therapy and specific drugs be reserved for those at truly high risk.

Summing Up

• High blood cholesterol increases the risk of a heart attack, but people over the age of sixty do not need to be as concerned about moderate elevations (250 to 260 mg/dL, for example) as a younger person.*

● Foods labeled "cholesterol-free" are not necessarily appropriate for a low-cholesterol diet, especially if they are high in palm and/or coconut oils.

● Cutting out excess calories and reducing intake of saturated fats may be as or more important than reducing consumption of foods high in cholesterol itself (like shrimp and so forth).

● People with high blood pressure should do everything possible to keep cholesterol levels as close to normal as possible.

*A low-saturated-fat, low-cholesterol, moderately high soluble-fiber diet should be the mainstay of therapy unless lipid (fat) levels remain above 280 in persons with no other risk factors or above 260–265 in persons who smoke or have hypertension or diabetes, specifically if they are males under the age of 60 to 65 years.

13

SPECIAL PROBLEMS OF HYPERTENSION IN WOMEN

Men and women have almost an equal risk of having high blood pressure, but for women, there can be special problems, as illustrated by the following situation.

A thirty-three-year-old woman came to see me not long ago. Mrs. J. had been married for several years, and she and her husband very much wanted a baby. After two years of trying, she was finally about two months pregnant. The week before, she had visited her obstetrician, who found that her blood pressure was 150–170/100. He warned her of the dangers of hypertension to both her and her baby and had advised her that perhaps she shouldn't continue the pregnancy.

"We've been trying for this baby a long time," she said tearfully. "And if we don't have it now, we probably never will." She and her husband obviously didn't want to jeopardize her life or, on the other hand, risk having an unhealthy baby. Yet they didn't want to accept the fact that there was no option other than an abortion.

Unfortunately this woman's dilemma has become more common. In the last twenty or thirty years obstetricians have become more and more concerned about the possible complications of so-called high-risk pregnancies. Diseases such as diabetes or high blood pressure can carry an increased risk of miscarriages, stillbirths, and fetal abnormalities. There is also an increased risk to the mother. While these complications and possible poor outcomes are not the fault of the obstetrician in most instances, many physicians are reluctant to take on *any* patient who may pose special risks for the simple reason that they are concerned about being sued for malpractice. Thus, some may recommend that a woman avoid pregnancy or have an abortion rather than take a chance, even if the chance is small or complications can be avoided by proper treatment. As one of the obstetricians at my hospital said recently, "Why risk a malpractice suit if you know in advance that there may be a problem?" This tendency to practice medicine with an eye over the shoulder for a waiting lawyer may occasionally lead to depriving a patient of proper care. I can sympathize with my obstetrician colleagues. It's a major dilemma with no easy answer.

Of course, the counterargument in this particular situation is that we do have the ability to prevent many of the complications associated with hypertension during pregnancy. So long as the woman understands the possible risk and is willing to work with her doctor to keep her blood pressure under control, she has an excellent chance of having a healthy baby with little risk to herself. Great strides have been made in recent years in controlling hypertension during pregnancy. This does not mean that the risks have been eliminated, but more than ever, a hypertensive woman today can look forward to having a normal, healthy baby. It is a good idea, however, for her to be cared for either by an obstetrician experienced in treating hypertension during pregnancy or by an obstetrician working in collaboration with another physician who is knowledgeable in this area.

I reassured Mrs. J. that with proper treatment of her high blood pressure, she could anticipate a normal pregnancy and, most important, a healthy baby. In her case her blood pressure was controlled with small daily dosages of a diuretic and a beta-blocking drug. At first her obstetrician was very concerned about the use of any medication, especially a diuretic, during pregnancy. But we were able to show him several excellent scientific studies in which it had been demonstrated that with pregnant women who also have hypertension, good control of high blood pressure with low doses of these drugs did not harm the fetus. In fact, their use increased the chances of these women having normal babies.

Mrs. J.'s pregnancy progressed normally until she approached her last two weeks, when there was a moderate rise in her blood pressure. The obstetrician favored doing a cesarean section, but I felt that the baby would be better off if Mrs. J. could go to full term. Her medication was increased, and she went into labor on time. There were no significant problems, and happily she had a perfectly healthy six-and-a-half-pound girl. When I last saw her, Mrs. J. was enjoying motherhood, and her blood pressure was normal, as she had continued to take her medication. Over the years I have treated many such patients with similarly good results.

Only about 5 to 10 percent of pregnancies are complicated by high blood pressure. Basically there are two types of hypertension during pregnancy: (1) that which exists before pregnancy or develops during the first few months (Mrs. J. had this type) and (2) high blood pressure which develops in the fifth, sixth, or seventh month of pregnancy. This is the type of hypertension which is associated with toxemia of pregnancy.

Preexisting or Early Hypertension

Somewhat different standards are used when it comes to the diagnosing of hypertension during pregnancy. Normally, blood pressure decreases during the course of pregnancy, especially in the first three or four months. If a woman's usual blood pressure is 120/80 before she becomes pregnant, it will remain at these or *lower levels* until the last trimester. This decrease is the result of dilation of blood vessels throughout the body. If blood pressure is higher than 130–135/85–90 early in the pregnancy, it suggests a diagnosis of hypertension. (Although this may be a normal level in a nonpregnant woman, it is not normal during pregnancy.) If pressure is above these levels, it implies that primary hypertension is present and that it is not specifically related to the pregnancy. If, however, blood pressures remain between 100/70 and 120/80 during most of the pregnancy, then rise above 135–140/85–90 during the last two or three months, a diagnosis of pregnancy-related hypertension is justified. If there is swelling of the ankles or around the eyes, and if protein is found in the urine, toxemia of pregnancy is the likely cause.

Treatment During Pregnancy

Ever since the thalidomide tragedies of the late 1950s and early 1960s, when babies with serious congenital defects were born to women taking this mild tranquilizer, both physicians and women have been reluctant to use any medications during pregnancy. Virtually every substance the woman takes into her body during pregnancy crosses the placental barrier and may affect the baby as well as the mother. Thus, when a woman smokes a cigarette or drinks an alcoholic beverage, the developing baby is exposed to nicotine or alcohol. (Obviously we would not knowingly give a baby or young child a puff on a cigarette or a swig of alcohol.) Since the fetal liver is not developed enough to detoxify such substances properly, they may be particularly harmful to the baby. Fortunately, in the majority of cases, exposure to these substances does not produce lasting harm, but there are exceptions. Babies born to women who smoke are often smaller than average.

A similar argument is often made about taking any medication during pregnancy. There are, however, some important considerations. With medications the benefits must be weighed against the possible risks. If a medication is being taken to counter insomnia, as in the case of thalidomide, or just to make a woman less nervous, then the risks to the fetus may well outweigh the benefits. There are other cases, however, in which the risk of the mother's *not* taking the medication may well be greater than the risk of the drug itself. Hypertension is an excellent example. There is no question, in my opinion, that uncontrolled high blood pressure is a greater risk to both the fetus and the mother than taking antihypertensive medication. Of course, some drugs are safer than others, and in the treatment of any medical condition during pregnancy, the lowest possible dosage of the safest drug available should be given to manage the problem.

The 1988 report of the Fourth Joint National Committee on Detection, Evaluation and Treatment of High Blood Pressure summarizes the latest scientific consensus about the treatment of hypertension in pregnancy. To quote the report:

Hypertension during pregnancy may represent the syndrome of preeclampsia (pregnancy-induced hypertension) or chronic (essential) hypertension. In either situation, treatment of hypertension is beneficial in reducing both maternal and fetal mortality. *Therapy instituted before pregnancy may be con-*

tinued in hypertensive women who become pregnant. In women with preeclampsia, modified bed rest and proper diet may reduce the blood pressure satisfactorily. If not, antihypertensive drug therapy should begin (my italics).

Many obstetricians are reluctant to prescribe beta blockers, diuretics, and certain other antihypertensive medications during pregnancy. Here, too, the 1988 committee report was quite specific:

Methyldopa and hydralazine have been used extensively in pregnant women, but recent clinical studies indicate that beta-adrenergic blocking drugs also are effective in controlling blood pressure and improving fetal survival. Angiotensin-converting enzyme (ACE) inhibitors have been demonstrated to increase fetal mortality in pregnant animals and should probably be avoided during pregnancy. The calcium channel blockers have proven effective in controlling severe hypertension in late pregnancy, but they could cause a decrease in uterine contractions during labor.

As for the use of diuretics, the committee did not take a specific stand other than to note that in instances of preexisting high blood pressure in which the woman has been under successful treatment, the therapy should continue. I agree with the national report on this point, and I strongly advocate that the woman be continued on her medication, although perhaps at a lower dosage. Some physicians believe that drugs should be discontinued and restarted later if blood pressures rise. Since pressures normally decrease during pregnancy, this approach should be considered, but it should be remembered that maintaining normal blood pressures during the first few months of pregnancy is particularly important. If medication is stopped, blood pressures should be checked frequently, and if they rise to 130/80–85 or higher, medications should be restarted. If blood pressure remains within normal limits after the first trimester, we can sometimes reduce medication and still maintain normal pressures. However, if there is a subsequent rise in blood pressure, the dosage should be increased. In my experience, normal blood pressures have been maintained in most pregnancies in which the women have preexisting hypertension by having them continue their previous medications at somewhat reduced dosages.

There has been a great deal written in the medical literature regarding the possible dangers of using a diuretic during pregnancy. Many of these reports have been based on studies that I consider flawed. Specifically these studies suggest that a diuretic may decrease blood flow to the placenta, thereby compromising fetal blood supply and resulting in a smaller than expected baby. Yet it is well known that women who are hypertensive will often have small babies, regardless of whether or not they take diuretics or any other drugs. (The placentas often show numerous clots and shrunken areas, which result in less blood supply to the fetus and less growth.) Large-scale studies have not demonstrated a decrease in fetal survival among women treated with diuretics during pregnancy, and in my opinion, these medications can safely be used (in small doses) to control hypertension during pregnancy.

Still, there are many instances in which diuretics have been overused. For example, for many years pregnant women were placed on diuretic therapy for ankle swelling. This is no longer done; it is now accepted that ankle swelling is a normal aspect of pregnancy, especially during the last two or three months, when the enlarged uterus presses on the abdominal veins and hinders the return of blood from the legs back to the heart. The problem is related more to simple gravity than to a physical abnormality. For example, if you wear a tight garter or band around the thigh, your ankles may swell. Similarly, you might notice ankle swelling after a long airplane trip in which you have been sitting quietly for a long period with your legs lower than the rest of the body. Clearly, diuretics are not indicated in these situations. The same is true about giving diuretics to counter normal ankle and leg swelling in pregnancy. Initial overuse of diuretics and warnings about this may account for some of the reluctance among today's obstetricians to prescribe diuretics during pregnancy. Even so, warnings about dangers to the fetus, which in my opinion have not been adequately proved, undoubtedly account for much of the reluctance among obstetricians to prescribe these medications. While I heartily concur that diuretics should not be used for normal swelling, I believe that they still have a place in the treatment of hypertension in a pregnant woman, especially if she had been taking one of them before she became pregnant. The benefit would appear to outweigh any theoretical risk. As with all medications used during pregnancy, the dosage should be kept as low as possible and potassium levels in the blood should be checked more frequently during pregnancy than at other times.

Toxemia of Pregnancy

The second type of hypertension encountered during pregnancy is part of the complex referred to as toxemia of pregnancy or preeclampsia. Preeclampsia occurs in about 3 to 5 percent of pregnancies, most often in the last trimester, but it can develop anytime between the twentieth week and the first week after delivery. It is most common among women who are pregnant for the first time. The risk also is increased among women carrying two or more fetuses.

Preeclampsia is characterized by high blood pressure—a reading of 140/90 or higher, or a rise of 30 mmHg in systolic pressure and 15 mmHg in diastolic pressure (compared with prepregnancy readings)—protein in the urine, and swelling of the face and hands. Often the first sign a woman notices is puffiness around her eyes or tightness of a ring.

An example of preeclampsia is the case of Mrs. L. R., a healthy twenty-two-year-old who was pregnant with her first baby. During her first checkup her blood pressure was about 120/80; on the second and third visits it had decreased to 110/70. In the fifth month it had risen to 135/80, and by the seventh month it was 140/90—clearly a sign of evolving preeclampsia. Her obstetrician ordered bed rest for one week and lying on the left side, which has been found helpful in many patients, but there was no decrease in blood pressure. Even with continued bed rest, her blood pressure rose to 150/100. She also had facial puffiness and ankle swelling. At that point her obstetrician referred Mrs. L. R. to me.

She was started on a small dosage of a beta blocker, and within a week her blood pressure was back to a normal 130/80. She continued on the beta blocker for the rest of her pregnancy and was delivered of a normal baby. Perhaps bed rest for the remainder of her pregnancy would have produced similar results, but it is difficult for an active, otherwise healthy woman to

spend six or eight weeks in bed. And there is no guarantee that this will eventually reduce blood pressure
and prevent worsening preeclampsia. A low-dose beta
blocker or any one of several other antihypertensive
drugs seems like an easier and more exacting approach
to reducing blood pressure. Some obstetricians are
concerned that a beta blocker given to the mother may
slow down the fetal heartbeat too much. While this is a
theoretic possibility, studies in Scotland and England
have demonstrated that these drugs cause no apparent
harm to the baby.

The precise causes of preeclampsia are unknown,
but researchers believe it is related to a substance or
substances in the placenta that interfere with normal
regulation of blood pressure. Normally the body's
usual response to adrenalinelike substances is lessened
during pregnancy. But women who develop toxemia
seem to be more sensitive to these substances. In addition, it is believed that there may be a defect in the
production of certain hormones or prostaglandins that
regulate the dilation of blood vessels. If these are decreased, narrowing or constriction of the vessels occur.
Reduced kidney function may result, with retention of
salt and water and with swelling. (Some researchers are
studying the use of *small* doses of aspirin to prevent
preeclampsia because of the known effect of aspirin on
the prostaglandin system.)

In the past untreated toxemia often led to premature birth or even the death of the fetus and sometimes
the mother as well. It is understandable that women
who have heard horror stories of the consequences of
toxemia may feel panicked at such a diagnosis. Panic
and fear in themselves can exacerbate the condition.
All women should be aware of the warning signs of tox-

emia, especially if they are pregnant for the first time or have histories of high blood pressure. But they also should know that toxemia almost always can be handled successfully.

There are two general approaches to treating toxemia. One calls for almost complete or modified bed rest as soon as the symptoms appear. In some medical settings the woman is actually hospitalized for four to eight weeks and is delivered by cesarean section just before full term. Statistics documenting the success of this approach are impressive, but for most women the treatment is probably more rigid than is required. The long hospitalization or lengthy bed rest at home can place a psychological burden on all concerned, even if the results are good. It can also be costly, both in medical bills and in lost work time.

The approach followed for Mrs. L. R. is more practical than prolonged bed rest and may be equally successful. I advocate some bed rest—an afternoon nap and several rest periods during the day if at all possible. If a woman is still working, she might try to cut her schedule to half time or work out breaks during which she can lie down. Simply lying on the left side helps alter blood flow to the kidney and placenta and increases the output of urine. The woman should be encouraged to drink plenty of water. I advocate mild sodium restriction, although there is medical disagreement on this point. Some experts believe it does little good and may even worsen the condition. However, this has not been my experience.

I also advise using beta blockers or other antihypertensive drugs to lower the blood pressure. It is important to lower the blood pressure to prevent further blood vessel injury and decreased blood flow to the placenta. The diminished blood flow can result in a baby with a low birth weight and other problems. In preeclampsia, diuretics generally are not recommended, although I and others have used them without any specific harmful effects to the fetus or the mother.

In some unusual cases the preeclampsia may progress to a much more severe stage known as eclampsia. This is usually characterized by extremely high blood pressure, seizures, blood-clotting abnormalities, and, if it is untreated, coma and even death. Eclampsia may usually, but not always, be prevented by earlier detection and treatment of preeclampsia. I vividly recall one case in which I was called by a nurse to the hospital emergency room. There I found a twenty-nine-year-old woman whose pregnancy was near term. She was having convulsions, her blood pressure was 230/130, and she was suffering from momentary respiratory arrest, during which time she stopped breathing altogether.

I learned that the woman had experienced progressively rising blood pressures of 140–160/90–100 during the previous two or three months. As noted earlier, ordinarily these readings might not be considered exceptionally high, but during pregnancy they are warning signs that should be taken seriously. She had been treated with bed rest alone, partially out of her obstetrician's fear of administering any medication to lower her blood pressure. Unfortunately hers was one of the cases in which bed rest was ineffective, and antihypertensive medications should have been used to prevent the kind of crisis we were now witnessing. At this point the obstetrician was *still* reluctant to start aggressive therapy to lower her blood pressure, other than giving magnesium sulfate, an

Other Special Problems:

BIRTH CONTROL PILLS AND HYPERTENSION

Mrs. L. M., a healthy twenty-seven-year-old, was referred to me because of high blood pressure that was not responding as well to medication as her doctor thought it should. She had been on treatment for four years, was not overweight, and her blood and urine tests were normal.

"Are you taking any medications other than what your doctor has prescribed for your blood pressure?" I asked her.

"No, Doctor," she said. "I'm very healthy and hardly ever take even an aspirin."

I noted that she had been married for six years but had no children. "Do you use any method of birth control?" I asked.

"Why, yes," she replied. "I've been on the pill for years."

Like many people, Mrs. L. M. did not consider birth control pills a form of medication. In fact, they are drugs that can affect many body systems. For reasons we do not fully understand, they may cause high blood pressure in a very small number of women who use them. The most susceptible are women with genetic tendencies to develop hypertension or those who are overweight. The hormones in the pill promote salt and water retention, and some researchers believe that this accounts for the rise in blood pressure among susceptible women.

If the high blood pressure develops shortly after a woman has started an oral contraceptive, the association of the two is more apparent. But sometimes we see women like Mrs. L. M. who have used the pill for years and then are noted to have high blood pressure. In such cases physicians may not make the connection.

After explaining to Mrs. L. M. that her birth control pills might well account for her high blood pressure, I advised her to switch to another form of contraception to see if this would make a difference.

She agreed to go off the pill. I also decided to stop her antihypertensive medication for the time being to see if stopping the pill would be sufficient to lower her blood pressure. When I saw her four months later, her blood pressure was again in the normal range. This does not always happen, but quite often simply stopping the pill will be enough to reduce blood pressure. Actually contraceptive pills may be the most common form of "curable" hypertension among young women, even though it is relatively rare. Only a very small percentage of women on the pill develop high blood pressure because of the oral contraceptives, but the fact that many millions of women use this form of birth control means that the total number who develop hypertension is substantial.

Women who are hypertensive or who have other vascular problems are not advised to use oral contraceptives because of an increased risk of stroke. If blood pressure is normalized with treatment and the woman cannot find another acceptable form of contraception, the pill might be used, but blood pressure must be carefully monitored. Women who smoke probably should also not take oral contraceptives because of an increased risk of heart attack or stroke.

old standby of obstetricians that is not a very good blood pressure-lowering drug. It was obvious that without some specific treatment both the woman and her baby might die.

We started intravenous treatment, using a diuretic and a beta blocker. We later added a third drug, hydralazine, which helps dilate blood vessels. In less than an hour the convulsions stopped and blood pressure returned to near-normal levels. The woman was again able to breathe on her own. Twelve hours later a cesarean section was performed and a healthy baby was delivered. Some four years later the child is growing and developing normally. Although the mother has some residual weakness of an arm, she, too, is alive and well.

Obviously this is an extreme case, but it illustrates my point that it is much better to control blood pressure early, even if it means giving medication during pregnancy, than to allow hypertension and preeclampsia to progress to the point where a life-threatening emergency is precipitated. Today we rarely encounter this type of full-blown eclampsia, especially among women who have had regular prenatal care.

Unfortunately there are still women who have little or no prenatal care and show up at a clinic or emergency room with convulsions and blood pressures in excess of 200/100. There is a tendency to do an immediate cesarean section under these circumstances. While this may be less dangerous for the fetus, I would advocate trying to lower the blood pressure first since surgery is then less risky for the mother. This is not always possible, and an immediate cesarean section may be the only recourse. In such instances, removing the source of the toxemia—namely, the placenta—may be the only way to stop the symptoms of eclampsia.

Summing Up

• Hypertension per se is not a justification to avoid or terminate a pregnancy.

• The treatment of high blood pressure that is present before the onset of pregnancy, or develops within the first three to four months, is similar to that of a hypertensive patient who is not pregnant.

• Early detection and treatment of high blood pressure in pregnancy may prevent many of the complications associated with the disorder, including prematurity and babies with low birth weights.

• Appropriate antihypertensive medications given during pregnancy are probably not as harmful to the fetus as untreated high blood pressure.

• If toxemia of pregnancy develops with hypertension, usually in the last two to three months in a woman in her first pregnancy, medications should be used if bed rest is ineffective.

14

HYPERTENSION IN CHILDREN

Most cases of high blood pressure develop when people are in their thirties and forties, but there are instances of hypertension in children or adolescents. Childhood hypertension is relatively rare. The American Heart Association estimates that there are about two million youngsters six to seventeen years old with blood pressures that are higher than they should be. This is only a small fraction of the portion of adults who have high blood pressure. A specific cause is found in a much higher percentage of children than in adults, and hypertension can actually be cured in these cases. Fortunately, if we don't find a curable cause, we now have effective ways of treating childhood hypertension without affecting growth, development, or energy levels.

Normally children have lower blood pressures than adults; their levels increase as they grow older. For example, most babies have blood pressures of about 70–80/40–50, and by adolescence the typical readings will be about 110/70 or so (see Table 14:1.)

Detecting Childhood Hypertension

Ordinarily we doctors do not measure blood pressure in very young infants because to get truly accurate readings, we might have to insert a needle into an artery.

High blood pressure in infancy is very unusual, so unless there are specific problems, such as failure to grow normally, circulatory difficulties, or a behavioral pattern suggesting headaches, for example, we usually wait until the child is two or three years old to do the initial measurement. This, too, may be difficult to do accurately because the child may move or cry, and this will cause the pressure to go up. Thereafter routine pediatric checkups usually include a blood pressure measurement, although it's probably not necessary unless the initial readings at ages two and three are in the high or high-normal ranges. Blood pressures should be measured during early adolescence, at ages eleven, twelve, thirteen, and fourteen, and again in young adulthood.

Except in very unusual circumstances, there is little value in parents' trying to measure a child's blood pressure at home, especially if they use their own adult-size cuffs. There are different size cuffs, including very small ones for young children. Remember, a cuff that is too large may give readings that are lower than they really are. In general, the same guidelines are followed for diagnosing high blood pressure in children as in adults (See chapter 2). If the first reading is high, the child's blood pressure should be measured two or three more times during the visit.

Blood pressure should be measured in both arms on the first visit, and the pulse checked in the groin area. If pulses are decreased or absent, then blood pressure should be taken in the legs. If blood pressure is high in the arms, but low in the legs, a congenital abnormality called coarctation of the aorta may be present. In these cases the major artery that carries blood from the heart is narrowed just after it branches into the arteries that go to the brain and arms. Blood pressure is elevated in the upper part of the body but is low in the lower half. Typically the child will have strong pulses in his arms and weak or absent pulses in the legs. This rare condition is more common in boys than girls. It can be surgically corrected, thereby curing the problem and preventing subsequent enlargement of the heart or development of the blood vessel—changes of untreated hypertension. This diagnosis may be missed in childhood and picked up on a routine exam later on.

Sometimes the first reading during an office visit will be high, and one taken a few minutes later, after the child has calmed down, will be normal. However, if the average of three readings taken during the course of an office visit is above normal, then an appointment for another examination should be made. As with adults, children whose blood pressures are high when measured in the doctor's office can be normal at other times. Or the blood pressure may be high on the first visit and then normal on subsequent visits. Two or three examinations are usually needed to establish a diagnosis unless, of course, the readings are very high or there are other symptoms to confirm a diagnosis of hypertension. It is important to note, however, that as in adults, we should not ignore these transient or temporary elevations of pressure. They are telling us something about the way the nervous system functions, and these children should have their blood pressures checked every six to twelve months.

Studies have found that children whose blood pressures fall in the high-normal ranges are more likely to go on to develop adult hypertension than are those in the middle or lower ranges. Since high blood pressure also has a strong hereditary tendency, particular attention should be paid to youngsters whose parents or other close relatives have hypertension.

TABLE 14:1
*Approximate Upper Limits of Normal Blood Pressure
According to Age of Child**

Age	Blood Pressure mm Hg
6 or younger	110/75
6 to 10	120/80
11 to 14	125/85
15 to 18	135/85–90

*If readings are above these levels, pressures should be rechecked.

Causes of Childhood Hypertension

Unlike the case with adults, high blood pressure in a child is more often caused by a specific disorder. This is especially true if the blood pressure is quite high or the child is under the age of ten to twelve. Thus, in the diagnosing of childhood hypertension, special tests that we doctors ordinarily do not need for adults may be justified. *The younger the child, the more likely it is that a curable cause of high blood pressure will be found.*

When I encounter a child with high blood pressure, I begin by looking for signs of organ damage, much as I would do with an adult. I also look for primary or specific causes of the high blood pressure; kidney disorders are among the more common of these. Clues can be found by listening for a murmur over the kidney arteries in the abdomen and by tests of the blood and urine, although kidney or blood vessel X-ray studies may be needed to identify the specific problem. Either an infection or a narrowing of one or both arteries that supply blood to the kidneys may be found. Treatment can then be directed to the cause of the elevated blood pressure. In the case of artery narrowing, surgery may be necessary.

Endocrine or hormonal disturbances also can cause childhood hypertension. I recently saw a six-year-old boy who was referred to me by an alert pediatrician because of persistent high blood pressure. In examining the child, I noticed that he was pale and sweating profusely, although the examining room was quite cool, and his blood pressure fluctuated between 140/90 and 220/110. These all were signs of too much adrenaline. In fact, further studies (a twenty-four-hour urine and CAT scan) confirmed that this child had an adrenal tumor that was excreting large amounts of adrenaline, the cause of his high blood pressure. Removal of the tumor corrected his problem.

Another endocrine disorder leading to hypertension is a rare condition called hyperaldosteronism, in which the adrenal glands secrete too much of the hormone called aldosterone. This hormone controls the body's sodium and water balance, and an excess can lead to retention of fluids and to high blood pressure. This condition can usually be diagnosed by blood tests, a twenty-four-hour urine test, and a CAT scan. If a specific tumor (which rarely, if ever, is malignant) is found, it can be removed. If just overactivity of the adrenal glands is found, medical therapy will usually control the blood pressure.

Some children develop a transient form of hypertension at about the time of their adolescent growth spurt. Pressures often return to normal when full growth is achieved, but they may remain in the high-normal range. The reasons for this adolescent hypertension are unknown; some researchers believe it is related to hormonal changes. Even if blood pressures return to normal, the child should be checked every year or two during young adulthood since studies have found that these individuals are more likely to develop primary hypertension at a later date.

Children who develop juvenile diabetes are at greater risk of developing elevated blood pressures, and they should be monitored regularly and treated if necessary. *It is extremely important to keep the blood pressures of diabetic patients at normal levels.*

Just how much testing is carried out to find the cause of childhood hypertension depends upon the age of the child and the severity of the disease. As noted, a young child with high blood pressure is more likely to have some other underlying disease; therefore, more extensive testing is justified. Very often there will be other symptoms or clues pointing to a possible cause. In contrast, an older child who has mildly elevated blood pressures is more likely to have early primary or essential hypertension, and extensive kidney or other studies may not be needed.

When to Treat Childhood Hypertension

If the high blood pressure is due to some other disease, such as a kidney or hormonal disorder, treating the underlying cause often will cure the hypertension. The treatment approach to mild or moderate hypertension in children where a specific cause is not found is not as clear-cut, and there is still considerable disagreement among doctors about when and how childhood primary or essential hypertension should be treated. Some physicians argue against prescribing antihypertensive drugs for children and adolescents on the grounds that they may well be on medication for fifty to sixty years or more, and we simply do not know the effects of such long-term usage. We do have data on drug effects for more than thirty years, but this is still a theoretic concern. We know that untreated hypertension at any age shortens life, so I would argue for the same commonsense approach to lowering high blood pressure in children that is advocated for adults.

Under this approach I would begin with a trial of nondrug therapy: reduced salt intake, weight loss if appropriate, and increased physical activity. If after several months of the patient's really trying to adhere to this program the blood pressures remain elevated, I recommend low doses of medication to lower the blood pressure. Beta blockers may be the drugs of choice in young people, especially adolescents with rapid pulse rates or pressures that vary considerably with changes in position. Typically, small dosages are sufficient (for example, 20 mg twice daily of propranolol, or 25 mg of atenolol or metoprolol). Side effects at these dosages are minimal, and the drugs are usually tolerated well. An exception might be the competitive athlete who may experience some fatigue on maximum exertion.

Diuretics also may be prescribed. Again, the dosages should be low (for example, 25 mg of hydrochlorothiazide every other day) and increased to higher levels (e.g., 25 mg daily) if blood pressures remain high. Occasionally a small dose of a beta blocker combined with a small dose of a diuretic will be necessary to keep blood pressures at normal levels.

There is some evidence that lowering elevated blood pressures in young people will help prevent progression to more serious levels during adulthood. Early control can also help solve other problems, such as the one encountered by one of my young patients. This particular young man, a nineteen-year-old college freshman with aspirations to continue his football career, was sent to me by his college coach. During his high school years his blood pressures had been mildly elevated to about 145/85. At that time both his coach and school physician decided he did not need treatment, and he was allowed to play.

By the time he tried out for his college team, his blood pressures had risen to 150–170/85–90, and the coach was reluctant to accept him on the team. I found him to be a well-built, muscular young man—five feet ten inches tall and weighing 195 pounds. As with most football players, he followed a rigorous weight lifting regimen to build muscle strength. His blood pressure was consistently elevated, but tests failed to reveal any evidence of an underlying cause for his hypertension. Actually it is not uncommon to see this kind of high blood pressure characterized mostly by systolic elevations in athletic young men. The questions are: (1) Should these people be treated and (2) should they be permitted to participate in competitive sports such as football?

I favor treating these young men in much the same way I outlined earlier for adolescents, with either a diuretic or a beta-blocking drug. In some cases a converting enzyme (ACE) inhibitor may be indicated, although these drugs are more expensive. In my experience, the majority of these young men can have their pressures lowered to within normal limits without too much difficulty.

Perhaps the more difficult question, not just for the young men but also for their families' and their coaches' peace of mind, is whether they should be permitted to participate in competitive sports. A good deal depends upon how high their blood pressures go during exercise. This can be determined by having the person hop up and down for five to ten minutes or push against a stationary object for one to two minutes. While these activities may not exactly replicate what happens during a football game, rowing event, or other competitive sport, it still gives an idea of how high the pressure goes during exercise. If the systolic pressure does not rise above 180–190, I see no reason why the young person cannot participate in a full athletic program. However, in the case of the football player, I did urge that weight lifting be limited because this tends to increase blood pressure and places increased strain on the heart. Of course, once blood pressure has been controlled (with or without medication), everyone feels better about allowing participation, but even in these cases, wrestling or sports such as competitive rowing that require a great deal of straining against resistance (playing guard or tackle in football is another example) might be discouraged.

Some extremely vigorous sports that require tremendous exertion in a short period of time—for example, sprinting—may also not be a good choice. Basketball, tennis, soccer, or even long-distance running would probably be preferable.

With the young man described above, I recommended that his blood pressure be checked periodically, preferably at the end of a practice session or a game. His systolic pressure remained below 170/90 after exercise, and he was advised to continue on beta blocker therapy. His athletic prowess was not affected by medication. In other situations I have had to change medication because some athletes have been slowed down by treatment.

Can Early Intervention Prevent Later Hypertension?

Since high blood pressure has a strong hereditary component, the question of whether early intervention is of special value to children of hypertensive parents is important. Frankly I don't know the answer to this question, although it is logical that adopting good habits that help keep blood pressure normal may be useful and certainly will not do any harm. There are some data from laboratory studies that restricting salt intake in rats with a genetic susceptibility to develop hypertension has a preventive effect. Whether this applies to humans is not known.

In any event, it is not a bad idea to suggest that all children be encouraged to limit salt, to exercise regularly, and to stay as thin as possible. This is all the more important if the parents have high blood pressure. For example, it's a good idea to keep the salt shaker away from young children lest they develop a craving for salt. There is no reason to add salt to baby food. Breast milk is lower in sodium than cow's milk—another good reason to breast-feed a baby if at all possible.

I also urge my hypertensive patients to avoid overfeeding their children. Both high blood pressure and obesity have genetic components, and an *overweight person of any age has an increased risk of developing hypertension.* Obesity also is closely associated with high blood cholesterol and diabetes. *As stressed in Chapter 5, an obese adolescent usually becomes an obese adult. An obese infant has a greater chance of becoming an obese adolescent.* It is important not to get in the habit of overfeeding a baby. Many parents make the mistake of thinking every cry and whimper are about food when cuddling or some other form of attention is really what the child wants. If every cry is answered with food, it doesn't take long for the baby to equate eating with attention and comfort. Obviously a baby should be fed enough for adequate growth and development. But the notion that chubbiness is a sign of good health is contrary to fact. A chubby baby is apt to grow into an inactive chubby child or adolescent and, finally, an obese adult who will spend his or her next forty to fifty years trying to become thin. Prevention is, once again, easier than treating a disease.

Children may be brought up on a nutritious, tasty diet without being deprived of anything. Many parents fear their children are not eating enough and constantly urge, "Clean your plate," or, "Have just two more bites and you can have some ice cream." Under normal circumstances a child will eat when he or she is hungry and stop when the appetite is sated. Food should not be used as a reward. If parents set the tone by allowing junk foods only on occasion and small portions of ice cream, cake, and cookies on occasion and by presenting a balanced diet for their children, the odds are that the children won't become obese. In some families with a strong genetic tendency toward obesity, a low-calorie, low-fat diet may have to be instituted at an early age in children to prevent their following in their mothers' or fathers' footsteps.

Exercise is also an important factor in a healthy head start on life, and it is doubly important for children at high risk for developing hypertension. Unfortunately many of today's children develop a TV habit early in life and would rather spend long hours watching the tube than walking, running, cycling, playing ball, and engaging in other active play. A number of recent studies have documented that on the whole, today's schoolchild is in poor physical condition. Adults may be jogging and exercising more, but their children are likely to be budding couch potatoes. If possible, children should be encouraged to join in their parents' exercise regimens or, more important, to find enjoyable physical activities of their own.

Summing Up

• Although relatively rare, hypertension does occur in children.

• High blood pressure in a young child is more likely to be caused by a specific known cause than in adults. The younger the child, the greater the possibility.

• Treatment to lower elevated blood pressure is important in children, and nondrug therapy should be tried first.

• A preventive approach for children with family histories of high blood pressure makes good sense, even if there is no absolute proof that this will prevent hypertension in later years. Staying thin and active and keeping away from salt and salty foods may be all that is necessary.

15

HYPERTENSION IN THE ELDERLY

How do we define *elderly*? It used to be that the age of sixty was considered old, and most of the information we have about the results of treatment of hypertension in the elderly use this age as a cutoff point. A better definition might be sixty to seventy-five, young elderly; seventy-five to eighty-five, middle elderly; and over eighty-five years of age, elder elderly. In any event, this is the fastest-growing segment of our population. By the year 2000 more than 15 percent of all Americans will be over sixty years of age, so we had better have a strategy for handling hypertension in this population if we are going to make the "golden years" more productive and healthy.

Blood pressure rises with age, at least for people living in Western industrialized societies. In less acculturated societies the blood pressures of sixty- and seventy-year-olds are essentially the same as in younger people. Among Americans over the age of sixty, up to 40 percent have blood pressures above 140/90, and about half of these (or 20 percent of the total) have blood pressures above 160/95. Men and women are about equally affected. Hypertension is more common among elderly blacks than whites, but the gap is not as wide as that between young blacks and whites.

In the past many people thought that high blood pressure in the elderly was a natural phenomenon, that older people needed increased pressure to supply sufficient oxygen to the brain and other vital organs. We now know that this is a myth.

Some researchers contend that increased blood pressures with aging is an adaptation to a loss of elasticity of the aorta and other large blood vessels. As the aorta becomes more rigid as a result of atherosclerosis, the heart must pump harder to move blood along to distant parts of the body, and blood pressure rises. While this is probably a factor in many older people, it should not be considered a normal aspect of aging. There is some loss in elasticity of blood vessels in all of us as we grow older, but changes severe enough to cause high blood pressure are not a universal phenomenon with aging. Actually a rigid aorta with arteriosclerosic changes may be the result of long-standing, perhaps undetected or inadequately treated high blood pressure.

Regardless of the cause of hypertension in the elderly (for many older people, as in the young, the cause remains unknown), it is now well documented that even mild to moderate elevations of blood pressure in older people are associated with an increased risk of strokes, heart attacks, and heart and kidney failure. We may not be as aggressive about lowering "high" blood pressure in an elderly patient if he or she doesn't respond easily to diet or antihypertensive drugs, but it should be emphasized that good blood pressure control is important at any age, and treatment should be attempted.

Nondrug treatment should be attempted first in the over-sixty population, as it is in younger patients. Occasionally nondrug treatment reduces blood pressure to a normal level. But behavioral changes, especially dietary restriction, may be more difficult for an older individual to bring about. Weight loss is especially difficult to achieve. A three- to four-month trial period of treatment without medication is justified unless pressures are very high. However, a rigid or highly restrictive program is not justified.

Unfortunately a large segment of our population and doctors alike remain unconvinced of the need to pay attention to high blood pressure among older people. A recent patient of mine, a sixty-nine-year-old retired teacher, had been referred to me by his family physician, who was uncertain whether to treat the patient's blood pressure, which was 145–155/90–95. The patient himself insisted that he was fine and didn't want to be bothered. "I've never felt better," he insisted.

He seemed in good shape, but there was evidence of a slightly enlarged heart and impaired kidney function. His blood pressure was indeed elevated (155/95), and because of this, along with signs of early organ damage, I recommended that he start some medication. He had come prepared with several articles he had copied from popular magazines. One advocated "natural" treatment with diet and relaxation. Another quoted the oft-repeated myth that a little high blood pressure is actually beneficial to an older person, and a third warned of potentially severe side effects from antihypertensive medications. It turned out that the latter was of the most concern to this patient.

His first wife had died some years earlier, and two years ago he had remarried. "Doctor, I thought sex and romance were a thing of the past," he confided. "But my wife and I are still like newlyweds. I'm not happy about going on medication that may affect all this."

It took a lot of talking to assure him that sexual problems occur in only a small percentage of patients taking blood pressure-lowering medication. And if problems do occur, we can almost always overcome them by changing the dosage or the type of medication. Thus assured, he started therapy—happily without problems. Unfortunately some physicians may not have the time or be willing to take the time to discuss the concerns of the patient. It may be easier to say, "Well, okay, you feel good, why rock the boat? Let's just see what happens." Three to four years later, when the patient may experience a complication or kidney function gets worse, then and only then are the forces of modern medicine mobilized to treat; often it's too late to have a meaningful impact on the patient's life. Of course, if a doctor is not convinced that early treatment is beneficial, he won't even try to persuade a patient to accept treatment.

Types of Hypertension in the Elderly

There are two types of hypertension in the elderly. The most common is similar to the high blood pressure seen in younger people, in which both the systolic and diastolic readings are elevated. The second is referred to as isolated systolic hypertension. In this type of hypertension, the systolic pressures may be as high as 200 or 210 mmHg, while the diastolic pressures are in the normal range of 70 to 80. In the past there was a tendency to discount elevated systolic readings, especially if the diastolic pressures were normal. Today we recognize that isolated systolic hypertension carries an increased risk of stroke and heart attacks and that it should be treated. Recent data from the Framingham Heart Study also suggest that a fair number of people with systolic hypertension actually had systolic and diastolic hypertension at a younger age and that perhaps early treatment might have prevented "old age hypertension."

Approaches to Therapy

Although older people today are generally in better health than in previous generations, there still are numerous physiologic or bodily changes that occur as we grow older. Some of these changes alter our approach to treating hypertension or make treatment more difficult. These changes include:

● *Decreased heart function.* As we age, the heart beats less forcefully, resulting in a reduced amount of blood being pumped out with each contraction.

● *Decline in kidney function.* With age the number of filtering units in the kidney decreases. Even in the absence of diabetes, hypertension, or other disorders that affect the kidney, there may be a 40 to 50 percent decline in kidney function by the time we reach sixty or seventy. Fortunately for all of us, kidneys that are functioning at this level are still efficient enough to get rid of waste products. If hypertension or diabetes is present, however, kidney function deteriorates more rapidly, and kidney failure can occur. Waste products back up, and a disease called uremia may result.

● *Decline in liver function.* The liver serves as the body's chemical processing plant—a complex and monumental task. As we age, the liver's metabolic processes slow down and change. These changes are especially pronounced in a person who has consumed alcohol for many years or someone who has had chronic hepatitis or other liver disorders. Even lifelong teetotalers who have never had a liver disorder will experience some changes in liver function over the years. As a result, older people metabolize or handle many substances, including medications, more slowly than or differently from a younger person. In older persons certain drugs may not be tolerated well, and dosages may have to be adjusted. The older the person, the more important is this aspect of treatment.

• *Slowed body reflexes.* Many older people complain of feeling dizzy or light-headed when they suddenly change positions, such as standing after sitting or when getting out of bed in the morning. They also may experience spells of light-headedness or even fainting when they stand up in a warm room especially after a drink or two or a heavy meal. Normally when a younger person stands up suddenly, reflexes signal the heart to beat faster, and blood vessels in the abdomen or legs constrict or narrow so that more blood is made available to the brain. Symptoms may occur in older persons because it takes longer for the sensors in the vessels in the neck or near the aorta to signal the heart and blood vessels to ensure that the brain gets a steady supply of blood. In a younger person the changes are almost instantaneous, but an older person may require more than just a few seconds before the body makes the necessary adjustments. Instead of blood flow being maintained in the brain as it is in a younger person, the blood will tend to pool in the abdomen or legs of an older person. In some cases this pooling of blood in the lower extremities can lead to fainting.

Because of these physiologic changes, some physicians are extracautious or even reluctant to treat high blood pressure in an older person. They argue, for example, that it is often difficult to arrive at a proper drug dosage. In addition, many older people are already on medication for other conditions that may conflict with blood pressure-lowering drugs. For example, many of the drugs used for arthritis reduce the effectiveness of some of these medications. Because of reduced reflexes, drugs such as the vasodilators may increase the likelihood of fainting in some elderly patients.

While these are legitimate concerns that must be taken into consideration when treating hypertension in the elderly, they are not sufficient reasons to forgo treatment. Obviously these factors may influence the types of drug and the dosages that are used. In practice most older patients seem to tolerate medication fairly well, and in two large clinical studies—the Hypertension Detection and Follow-up Program Study (HDFP) and the European Working Party Study on Hypertension in the Elderly—the number of adverse reactions were not any greater in older individuals than in the trials in younger people. But you have to be careful. In my own experience several problems specific to the elderly include:

• *Loss of too much sodium following the use of a diuretic—with weakness, nausea, cramps, and other symptoms.* This is rare but should be watched for.

• *Excessive lowering of blood pressure in the standing position.* That's why blood pressure should be taken and followed in the upright position in older people.

Benefits of Treatment

A number of extensive and well-documented medical studies have demonstrated the value of treating hypertension in older people. Specifically, studies in Australia and Europe, and the Veterans Administration in the 1960s and the HDFP study in the United States have reported a significant decrease in strokes, heart failure, and overall deaths from heart and vascular disease in treated patients. In these studies diuretics, with or without a drug that protects against potassium loss, were used as initial treatment with other medications (beta blockers or centrally acting drugs) being added if necessary.

In fact, the specific drugs that are probably the most effective in older people are the diuretics and calcium channel blocking agents. Beta-blocking drugs may be somewhat less effective. Even so, normal blood pressure will result in a high percentage of cases when this class of drugs is added to a diuretic in patients who have not responded to a single drug. Still, blood pressure control in older persons is not achieved as easily or as often as in younger patients. In a recent study, for example, in my own patients, more than 80 percent of patients under sixty years of age achieved normal blood pressure readings with treatment, compared with about 70 percent among the sixty-plus group. At least part of these differences may be attributed to the fact that side effects in some older people may limit the *amount* of medication that can be used.

As noted, in general, severe reactions to medications do not appear to be any more common or more pronounced among older patients than younger ones, but there are more exceptions to the rule. Medications should be introduced at lower dosages and increased over a longer time period in the elderly. If this is done, there should be fewer problems. "Start low and go slow" is a good rule in the adjusting of dosages.

Economics may play a specially important role in how well blood pressure is controlled in the elderly. I remember one patient whose blood pressure was under good control in the early months of therapy, but then it began to climb back up. I tried increasing the dosage but with little effect. I suspected that this person might not have been taking the full dosage of medication. A check with the pharmacy revealed that he had not renewed his prescription on time, but when I asked him if he was out of pills, he said he still had plenty. In fact, he brought his pill bottle with him, and indeed, it was still half full. Further questioning revealed that instead of taking his pills twice a day as prescribed, he was only taking them in the morning.

"I don't really need the medication when I'm sleeping, do I?" he explained. "And it costs so much to have the prescription filled. This way I can save money and make the pills go twice as far."

This reasoning, however faulty, is not uncommon. Many older people, especially those on limited budgets or Social Security, will try to make their pills go farther by taking less than the recommended dosages. This may lead to an inadequate or poor response. If this is a problem, don't be afraid or embarrassed to discuss it with your doctor. Many times a physician can adjust the cost of medication by choosing less expensive drugs and using generic equivalents if these are available. Sometimes, of course, this will not be possible. More expensive therapies may be required to lower blood pressure. If an older person truly has difficulty paying for needed medication, there are a number of programs that can be of help. The AARP (American Association for Retired Persons) has a low-cost plan, and some pharmaceutical companies will provide free medication to people who cannot otherwise afford it. Local and state agencies also have programs to help pay for medication. You can check with your area office on aging to find out what if any service is available in your community.

As noted in Chapter 7, some antihypertensive medications are considerably more expensive than others that may be equally effective. Too frequently doctors fail to consider their patients' pocketbooks when prescribing medication.

Systolic Hypertension

Heretofore we have concentrated on the treatment of ordinary primary hypertension (where both the systolic and diastolic levels are elevated) in the elderly. Isolated systolic hypertension is even a more common problem in people over sixty. Until recent years systolic hypertension was largely ignored unless the readings were very high, and to date, there are still no studies to document the benefit of treating "isolated" systolic blood pressure (for example, 160/70 to 200/80) in an elderly patient. But as already noted, there *is* evidence to support the fact that systolic hypertension is a major risk factor for heart and blood vessel problems. Long-term epidemiological studies indicate that systolic hypertension is just as much a risk factor for strokes, heart attacks, and heart failure as diastolic blood pressure elevation. Thus, even though we lack concrete evidence that lowering the pressure prolongs life, we support treating systolic hypertension if the pressure is above 160 mmHg, even though the diastolic readings are normal—*provided that it can be done simply and without causing too many side effects.* A preliminary study (the Systolic Hypertension in the Elderly study) demonstrated that blood pressure can be lowered in a high percentage of older persons with systolic hypertension by the use of a diuretic. A five- to seven-year study is presently under way to determine if this will reduce the occurrence of heart failure and strokes. My own experience suggests that it is more difficult to reduce isolated systolic blood pressure elevations to normal than it is to treat other types of hypertension. For example, fewer than 50 percent of my elderly patients with this finding had their pressures reduced to below 140/90 while about 70 percent of those with systolic/diastolic pressures in the sixty and over age-group were successfully treated.

A Final Word to the Naysayers

Invariably, when I talk about the benefits of treating high blood pressure in the elderly, someone will describe an aged uncle or acquaintance whose blood pressures are "through the roof." What's more, he or she may drink, smoke, weigh too much, and rarely move from in front of the TV set except to go to the refrigerator for another beer. And the kicker will be: "He's ninety-two and still going strong." This reminds me of Winston Churchill's gloating over the fact that he was fat, sedentary, smoked constantly, and drank a good deal but still reached an enviable old age. Yes, there are exceptions.

There are individuals who can break all the rules and live long lives even if they have multiple risk factors. Similarly, there are people who don't smoke or drink, exercise regularly, eat all the right foods, and still die young of heart attacks. There are exceptions on both ends of the spectrum. When we talk about risk factors, we are referring to population averages, not to a specific individual's odds. When we suggest that you remain thin, refrain from smoking, exercise, and lower your blood pressure, we are merely attempting to shift the odds in your favor and delay the onset of heart or blood vessel disease.

Summing Up

• Untreated mild to moderate elevations of blood pressures in older people are associated with an increased risk of strokes, heart attacks, and kidney failure.

• Both types of hypertension in the elderly (systolic and diastolic, and isolated systolic) are risk factors for heart and blood vessel problems and should be treated.

• The usual nondrug treatments should be tried first, but these solutions may not be successful in lowering blood pressure.

• Studies report a significant decrease in deaths from heart and vascular disease in older patients with systolic and diastolic hypertentension whose blood pressure has been lowered.

• As a general rule, blood pressure-lowering medication should be introduced at lower dosages and increased over a longer time period with elderly hypertensive patients.

16

PUTTING IT ALL
IN PERSPECTIVE

In my forty-plus years as a physician I have wit-
nessed major changes in the practice of medicine. It has
progressed from an era where few treatments were available for many of our most common illnesses to one
where there are any number of effective treatments available for patients with arthritis, diabetes, cancer, hypertension, and heart disease. It has progressed from an era
where diagnostic capabilities were limited to a time when
CAT scans, and magnetic resonance imaging can probe
for the smallest changes in almost any tissue and sur-
geons can transplant kidneys, lungs, and even hearts.
The medical profession has changed from a cottage industry of individual physicians who took care of patients
to a major industrial complex of technology and for-
profit hospitals that advertise for patients and offer in-
centives to doctors to use their facilities. It has fostered
the entrepreneurial physician who advertises his wares
like the traveling medicine man of yesteryear. All these
changes have obviously not been for the better, but some
have served to increase the length and quality of life for
millions of people. There is no better example of this
than the advances that have occurred in the treatment of
high blood pressure. Most important, in this instance the
benefits of the improvement in care have largely been
achieved without the use and expense of a high-tech
approach.

In previous chapters today's management of this once insidious and highly lethal disease has been put into perspective. A straightforward and simple approach to hypertension management works in most instances, hospitalization is rarely necessary, and effective treatment prolongs lives. Just the halving of stroke deaths in a single generation is in itself a tremendous achievement, one that American medicine can point to with considerable pride. There are still problems to be solved, but it is exciting to realize that a diagnosis of high blood pressure no longer implies an early disability or death *or* that someone has to turn his or her life upside down to get better. We owe a great deal to the pioneering chemists who struggled with the formulae of diuretics, beta blockers, calcium blockers, converting enzyme inhibitors, vasodilators, and other medications, *and* to the researchers who helped evaluate their use. We can look forward to newer medications that will make it even easier for the patient and the doctor to control blood pressure. Although there still are a few patients who cannot be treated to normal levels, today's wide array of highly effective blood pressure-lowering medications has put such cases in a distinct minority.

Patients today are better informed about hypertension and its treatment largely as a result of programs such as the National High Blood Pressure Education Program and the efforts of the American Heart Association and other organizations. These organizations and all of us as individuals must continue to counteract the purveyors of false information and miracle cures. It is distressing to those of us who lived through the era before effective treatment was available to note that some of our patients are still influenced by the Dr. Xs, the "world-renowned nutritionists," who advocate treating high blood pressure with an assortment of high-dose vitamins, special enzymes, or tonics instead of (in their words) those "toxic drugs that poison your body." How long will it take the public to recognize that Dr. X usually owns or controls the company that sells the "natural treatment pills"? Vitamins and enzymes are fine; we all need a certain amount of these to survive, but let's not forget the past. After all, nondrug treatment was the only method of therapy in the 1930s and 1940s, when hypertension was indeed a leading killer disease. While all drugs may produce side effects in some people, the medications that have been discussed in this book are generally safe and effective; their use has saved lives.

My objective in writing this book has been to give you the information you need to judge for yourself whether you are receiving optimal treatment, and to evaluate the information you read about in magazines or hear on the radio or television. The single most important message is that *all hypertension, no matter how mild, should be treated.* There is no single treatment that works or is advised for all patients. Some may need only to lose weight, cut back on salt, and increase their exercise to be adequately treated. Others may need a single pill a day. Still others may require fifteen or twenty pills a day.

In any event, treatment should be kept as simple as possible. The increasing reliance upon technology and testing instead of sound medical judgment is one of the changes that disturbs me about the direction of American medicine. Unquestionably we still have the world's best medical care system, but we may be moving in the wrong direction. The growing threat of malpractice litigation and other economic factors have contributed to this use of overtesting and an increased reliance on technology instead of judgment. Undoubtedly some of our newer techniques *have* resulted in better patient care, but many are overused and have been accepted as routine without proof that patients are benefited. The media has also helped raise hopes about a new test, treatment, or medication which may be years away from perfection. This is why I have tried to explain in detail when a procedure is justified and when it may not be. In the medical world of the future, patients may have to serve as their own advocates on more and more occasions. Your doctor may not be as helpful as he has been in the past in guiding you through a treatment program because of some of the pressures that have been discussed. I hope you can use the information in this book as a basis for asking the right questions and helping in your own management of hypertension and other risk factors for heart disease.

Outlook for the Future

Despite the tremendous gains of recent decades, I have no doubt that we will witness even more advances in the prevention and treatment of high blood pressure and heart disease in the years to come. These are likely to involve some technological advances, newer medications, and better methods to bring about behavioral changes. I even look forward to a time when we will truly understand the cause or causes of high blood pressure. Once we know these, we should be able to devise even simpler and more effective treatments. It may be that future generations will study hypertension for its "historic interest," as they now study polio or typhoid fever.

Granted, some may scoff at such predictions as being overly optimistic or even an impossible dream. But then, I doubt that President Roosevelt's doctors had any inkling from 1940–1945 that in just a few years the kind of severe hypertension that resulted in the death of this world leader would become highly treatable.

GLOSSARY

ADRENALINE: a substance that stimulates the heart rate, constriction of blood vessels, etc.

ALDOSTERONE: a hormone from the adrenal gland that helps to regulate the amount of sodium retained by the body.

ALPHA-ADRENERGIC BLOCKER: A drug that lowers blood pressure by blocking certain nerve receptors on blood vessel walls.

ANEURYSM: A small blisterlike expansion of blood vessels. Aneurysms represent weak spots in arteries, which may rupture and cause bleeding (hemorrhage).

ANGINA PECTORIS: Chest pain resulting from a temporary shortage of oxygen to a portion of the heart. May be caused by a narrowed coronary artery.

ANGIOTENSIN CONVERTING ENZYME (ACE) INHIBITOR: A drug that blocks the formation of angiotensin, a substance that constricts blood vessels.

AORTA: The main artery of the body into which blood is pumped from the heart's major chamber, the left ventricle.

ARTERIOLES: The tiny blood vessels which pass blood from the arteries to the capillaries.

ARTERIOSCLEROSIS OR ATHEROSCLEROSIS: Terms used interchangeably to indicate hardening of the arteries.

Caused by fatty materials within the artery walls, which narrow the blood vessels.

AUTONOMIC NERVOUS SYSTEM: The "involuntary" nervous system which controls heart rate, constriction and dilation of blood vessels, temperature, and intestinal tract functions.

BETA BLOCKERS: A group of medications that lower blood pressure, probably by reducing the rate and force of the heartbeat and possibly by affecting an enzyme system that controls blood vessel constriction. Beta blockers may also be used in the treatment of angina pectoris.

BLOOD PRESSURE: Pressure exerted against the walls of the arteries.

BLOOD VOLUME: Total amount of blood circulating in the body.

BRUIT: a murmur heard over a blood vessel that is narrowed.

CALCIUM CHANNEL BLOCKER: A drug that partially blocks the movement of calcium into the walls of blood vessels, thereby dilating the vessels and helping to lower blood pressure. Also used in treating angina pectoris.

CARDIAC OUTPUT: The amount of blood pumped by the heart each minute.

CARDIOVASCULAR: Refers to heart ("cardio") and blood vessels ("vascular") i.e., diseases of the *cardiovascular* system.

CAT SCAN: A computerized X-ray examination.

CATECHOLAMINES: Hormones such as norepinephrine and epinephrine (adrenaline).

CHOLESTEROL: A fatty substance in the body that is necessary to produce certain hormones and other necessary products for cell survival. It is found only in animal products, such as milk, eggs, and meat. If too much is present in the blood, it may hasten or promote hardening of the arteries.

High-density lipoproteins (HDL cholesterol): That portion of circulating fat-protein that helps remove extra fatty material from blood vessels—the "good" cholesterol.

Low-density lipoproteins (LDL cholesterol): That portion of circulating fat-protein that usually accumulates within the walls of blood vessels—the "bad" cholesterol.

COARCTATION OF THE AORTA: A congenital constriction of the aorta that leads to elevated blood pressure in the upper body and lower pressure in the lower body.

COLLATERAL CIRCULATION: Alternative circulation of the blood through smaller vessels when a major vessel is narrowed or closed.

CONGESTIVE HEART FAILURE: A consequence of untreated hypertension or severe coronary artery disease. Fluid backs up and accumulates in the lungs, legs, or other tissues because the heart is unable to pump efficiently.

CORONARY: Refers to the heart. Coronary arteries are those arteries that supply the blood to heart muscle.

CORONARY ATHEROSCLEROSIS: Narrowing of the coronary arteries as a result of the accumulation of fatty deposits within the walls of the arteries. Often referred to as coronary heart disease.

DIASTOLIC BLOOD PRESSURE: Pressure recorded when the heart is resting in between beats. The lower of the two numbers recorded when an individual's blood pressure is taken.

DIURETICS: Medications that wash out sodium from the body and help reduce blood pressure. Also used to treat heart failure when too much fluid is retained. .

ECHOCARDIOGRAM: an instrument that uses a sonar wave technique to visualize various parts of the heart.

EDEMA: Swelling of parts of the body, usually the legs or ankles, as a result of excess fluid.

ELECTROCARDIOGRAM (ECG, EKG): Test conducted to reveal abnormalities of the heart. A graph records the electric activity of the heart muscle.

EPINEPHRINE AND NOREPINEPHRINE (commonly referred to as adrenaline): Hormones secreted by the adrenal glands that speed up the heart rate and raise blood pressure.

HYPERALDOSTERONISM: Excess production of the hormone aldosterone that results in high blood pressure, potassium loss, weakness, and the accumulation of excess sodium and fluid. A curable form of hypertension.

HYPERKALEMIA: An excess of potassium in the blood.

HYPERTENSION: Medical term for high blood pressure.

HYPOKALEMIA: A depletion of potassium in the blood.

HYPOTENSION: Medical term for low blood pressure.

LABILE HYPERTENSION: Unstable blood pressure. Pressure may be high at some times and normal at others.

MM HG (MILLIMETERS OF MERCURY): Refers to the height to which blood pressure pushes a column of mercury.

PALPITATION: A feeling of pounding or racing in the heart area. May be caused by a rapid or irregular heartbeat.

PHEOCHROMOCYTOMA: A tumor of the adrenal gland that causes an excess production of adrenalinelike hormones. A curable form of hypertension.

POSTURAL HYPOTENSION: Unusually low blood pressure when an individual stands up after sitting or lying down.

POTASSIUM: A mineral found in the cells of the body and in various foods. Needed by the body to maintain proper biochemical balance. Salt substitutes usually contain potassium.

PREECLAMPSIA: A medical term to describe a condition during the last three months of pregnancy. Characterized by fluid retention, high blood pressure, headaches, and other symptoms. Commonly referred to as toxemia of pregnancy.

PROSTAGLANDINS: Hormonelike substances that are important in a number of body processes, including nervous system functions, regulation of blood vessel size, and clotting mechanisms.

RENIN: An enzyme secreted mainly by the kidney which is important in regulating blood pressure.

SALT: Ordinary table salt is sodium chloride (NaCl).

SODIUM: A component of salt (about 40 percent of salt is sodium). A mineral that may contribute to high blood pressure if taken in large amounts by people who are sodium-sensitive. It is found naturally in many foods and also in baking soda, some antacids, MSG (monosodium glutamate), and certain food preservatives.

SPHYGMOMANOMETER: A device designed to measure blood pressure.

STROKE: Sudden loss of function in a part of the brain as the result of interference with its blood supply. May be caused by a clot (thrombus) or a rupture of a blood vessel (hemorrhage).

SYMPATHETIC NERVOUS SYSTEM: Part of the autonomic nervous system which, when stimulated, narrows blood vessels and causes a rise in blood pressure and so forth.

SYSTOLIC BLOOD PRESSURE: Pressure recorded at the time when the heart is contracted. The larger of the two numbers given in a blood pressure measurement.

TARGET ORGANS: Parts of the body such as the heart, brain, and kidney that may be damaged by untreated hypertension.

UREMIA: The result of kidney failure. Waste products accumulate in the body because the kidneys are unable to excrete them through the urine.

VASCULAR: Refers to blood vessels.

VASOCONSTRICTOR: An agent that causes constriction of blood vessels.

VASODILATOR: An agent that causes the arterioles to relax or dilate.

EPILOGUE

Since the publication of *Lower Your Blood Pressure and Live Longer* in 1989, there have been several important studies that have added to our knowledge about both the causes and treatment of hypertension and other risk factors for heart disease. However, a number of unresolved controversies remain. Many of these research reports and medical debates have received considerable media attention. As might be expected, some of these headline-grabbing stories have confused rather than clarified some issues. This epilogue is intended to put recent research reports into their proper perspective.

Borderline Hypertension

There is increasing evidence to support some treatment of even borderline high blood pressure, for example, blood pressures in the range of 135-145/85-90. One important study has confirmed that sustained blood pressure in this range, even in relatively young people, may increase the risk of target-organ damage. An increased thickening of the left side of the heart (left ventricular hypertrophy—L.V.H.) occurred in these individuals when compared to those whose pressures stayed within more normal limits or were lowered. L.V.H. is an important complication of high blood pressure because the thickening of heart muscle eventually reduces its ability to pump efficiently and also may increase the possibility of various heart rhythm abnormalities. The findings of this study do not suggest that persons with borderline high blood pressure require vigorous treatment, but supports measures to prevent a further rise in blood pressure, and perhaps steps to lower it into the normal range. Many of the interventions in this group of subjects involve nondrug treatment—especially weight loss if appropriate.

Dietary Treatment

Several recent research reports have described the possible role of diet in preventing high blood pressure. One of the most significant studies was published in January 1990. It involved more than 800 men aged 25 to 49 who had relatively normal blood pressures (diastolic readings below 90). The study participants were divided into several groups. Some were counseled on dietary changes intended to lose weight. Others were instructed to reduce their salt (sodium) intake, and others were counseled to increase potassium intake while reducing sodium and total calories.

At the end of three years, there had been only a 10 percent decrease in sodium (salt) intake, despite repeated efforts to reduce intake to a greater degree. There was only a 4 percent decrease in total weight, suggesting what many practitioners and patients know—sustaining a loss in weight is difficult, even in a somewhat controlled program.

All groups demonstrated minor reductions in blood pressures—about 2.5/2.0 mm Hg. The greatest decrease, however, was among those who lost weight. It is of interest that fewer people in this group progressed to high blood pressure than in the other groups. This is significant because most (if not all) hypertension specialists now believe that weight reduction is probably the most important dietary approach to preventing high blood pressure—and indeed, the most helpful nondrug intervention in treatment. Although the numbers in this study were not dramatic, they indicate that if people would lose excess weight and keep it off, it might be possible to prevent at least some individuals from becoming hypertensive.

Another recent study has assessed the effectiveness of treating mild high blood pressure with a combination of medication and diet. After six months, patients who were treated with blood pressure–lowering drugs and dietary intervention showed the lowest cardiovascular risk. In this study, the dietary component of treatment entailed weight loss as well as a low-sodium, high-potassium diet.

This new data adds to our body of knowledge regarding the benefits of nondrug management of hypertension. It should, however, be emphasized, that most people with elevated blood pressure still require therapy with drugs, but management may be simplified and be more effective if weight loss and salt reduction are part of the program.

Diabetes and High Blood Pressure

Dietary studies take on added importance when we consider another cardiovascular risk factor—diabetes. As we have pointed out, this is more common in people with hypertension than in those with normal blood pressure. Recent studies associate obesity, defined as 15 percent to 20 percent above desirable weight, with an increased resistance to the effects of insulin. Insulin resistance means that the body is not able to adequately burn up or metabolize glucose (sugar)—its major fuel—at "normal" insulin levels, and an excess amount of insulin must be secreted by the pancreas. In time, the body may not be able to keep up the insulin supply, levels of blood sugar increase, and diabetes may develop. The combination of obesity and insulin resistance may also be accompanied by a reduction in protective (or good) HDL cholesterol, and an increase in LDL (or bad) cholesterol and triglycerides, another fatty substance that travels through the bloodstream.

The combination of low HDL cholesterol and elevated LDL cholesterol and triglycerides may be found in cases of high blood pressure, especially in obese hypertensive patients. Some researchers even suspect that hypertension may be a metabolic disorder linked to insulin resistance. In any event, these studies give still additional credence to recommendations that you stay as thin as possible, especially if you have a family history of diabetes, to possibly prevent diabetes and hypertension.

White-coat Hypertension

This term refers to blood pressure measurements that are elevated when taken in a doctor's office, but may be normal at home or at work—this was discussed briefly in Chapter 2. Several new reports have again questioned whether the elevated readings in the doctor's office should be considered as a guideline for treatment. I continue to disagree with suggestions that "white-coat hypertension" is not clinically significant. These blood pressure readings do indicate at least a tendency toward or the presence of hypertension. Although some patients will experience a rise in blood pressure due to the anxiety of having it measured by a doctor and then record normal levels at home or at work, the transiently elevated pressure should not be ignored. Physicians are being advised by some researchers to use 24-hour blood pressure monitoring to delineate the reactors from the persons whose pressures do not spike when they see their doctor. This expensive procedure adds little to a management program. As suggested, some blood pressures taken weekly at home, over time, may provide more valuable information at lower cost.

Safety of Diuretics

There have been numerous media reports suggesting that diuretics—one of the best and least costly medications used to treat high blood pressure—may actually increase the risk of a heart attack. Many of these reports and headlines followed the release of a four-month study of 50 patients by Swedish researchers which suggested that diuretics increase insulin resistance and may also raise cholesterol levels, and may therefore increase the risk of a heart attack. When the Swedish report first appeared in *The New England Journal of Medicine,* it garnered headlines—often on page one—in more than 200 United States newspapers. The story was also carried on national TV and radio news programs.

Actually, the report was not the fast-breaking news that the media attention suggested. It reiterated what physicians have known for many years (since the 1960s), namely, that diuretics do produce short-term elevations in blood cholesterol levels, and that the drugs may also increase insulin resistance and blood sugar. Most of these metabolic changes tend to be short-term and are probably of limited clinical significance. Long-term follow-up studies of patients taking diuretics have failed to show a major risk of persistently elevated blood sugar or the development of diabetes, except in a small number of cases (probably about 1 percent). The rises in blood cholesterol levels also tend to be transient. (See Chapter 7.)

In short, I still believe that diuretics should continue to be used as initial therapy in a large number of hypertensive patients, based on the drugs' long-term record of safety and effectiveness. They also are less costly than other antihypertensive medications—an important factor in this era of spiraling medical costs. Blood sugar and cholesterol levels should probably be checked within 3 to 6 months after a diuretic is started. If there is a dramatic change, more careful monitoring or a change in therapy may be indicated.

Benefits of Long-Term Treatment

The April 7, 1990 issue of *Lancet,* a leading British medical journal, analyzed a large number of clinical studies and once again affirmed the benefits of long-term treatment of hypertension. The analysis showed that patients whose high blood pressure had been treated for 3 to 7 years experienced more than a 40 percent decrease in strokes and stroke deaths and a 14 percent decrease in fatal and nonfatal heart attacks. This analysis of all of the major studies is important: there are still some doctors who maintain that, although the treatment of hypertension might reduce strokes and prevent heart failure or progression of mild to more severe hypertension, it has little effect on heart attacks.

I disagree with these doubters: early treatment of hypertension will, indeed, prevent many heart attacks and deaths from coronary artery disease. It is important to emphasize, however, as we do throughout this book, that high blood pressure is only one of several major risk factors for heart attacks, and a preventive program should also include smoking cessation, moderate exercise, and the lowering of blood cholesterol levels.

In addition to the *Lancet* report, there are interesting follow-up data from several large clinical treatment trials in the United States, including the Hypertension Detection and Follow-up Program (HDFP) and the Multiple Risk Factor Intervention Trial (MRFIT). After more than an 8-year follow-up period in the HDFP study, there is further evidence of a decrease in heart disease mortality; the benefit appears to be greater than that achieved at 5 years. This is also true of the MRFIT study. After

10.5 years, the reduction in cardiovascular disease in the vigorously treated compared to the less vigorously treated subjects is greater than it was at 5.6 years, suggesting that it may take time to actually detect some treatment benefits. The bottom line is that we have increasingly significant data affirming that the management of high blood pressure with medication (plus nondrug treatment) is beneficial and should be pursued in the majority of patients with high blood pressure, especially if they have other cardiovascular risk factors. Benefit clearly outweighs the possible risks of treatment.

New Antihypertensive Drugs

Over the past few years, a number of new antihypertensive drugs have been introduced, but none of these represents breakthroughs or major departures from past treatment strategies. (The newer drugs have been added to the lists in Chapter 7). Among the calcium blockers (see Chapter 7), several new brands have been approved for use in the United States. Some are reformulations of older drugs that have a longer duration of action, so that they can now be taken once a day. This, of course, is a major advantage and makes it easier for the patient to stay on medication. One of these medications, procardia XL, a long-acting formulation of nifedipine, appears to be as effective as the shorter-acting drug. It can now be taken in a single daily pill, and the side effects, such as ankle swelling, headaches, and palpitations, are less than with regular nifedipine.

New ACE (angiotension converting enzyme) inhibitors are being tested and should be on the market soon. These agents continue to grow in popularity with physicians; they are effective and have few side effects with the exception of a dry, hacking cough that we have now seen in about 10 to 15 percent of our patients. This cough, which is more common in women, may occur within the first month of therapy or has occasionally been noted after 4 to 6 months. It usually disappears after the drug is stopped and its long-term significance is unknown.

ACE inhibitors, in combination with diuretics, continue to be one of the most effective approaches to treatment of a large number of hypertensive patients who do not respond to a single medication.

Several new beta blockers have been introduced. (See chart in Chapter 7.) These may not have major advantages over previous beta blockers, but they do give the prescribing physician more options. There is also ongoing research on new drugs that block constrictor substances in different ways or have mixed mechanisms of action, such as dilating blood vessels directly while also blocking beta adrenergic receptors. There is no question that over the next 5 to 10 years, new types of antihypertensive drugs will become available, and hopefully, these will further improve and simplify the management of hypertension.

The Cholesterol Controversy

The importance of blood cholesterol continues to be a major source of controversy and confusion. One best-selling book (by a science writer, not a medical scientist) hypothesized that there is little or no scientific data to support the national drive to convince people to lower their blood cholesterol levels. He is clearly wrong. I continue to believe that there are sufficient experimental and epidemiological or population data linking elevated cholesterol levels to an increase in the risk of cardiovascular disease. I am not convinced, however, that giving cholesterol-lowering drugs to persons over the age of 65 to 70 is justified unless there are other risk factors present. A low-fat, low-cholesterol diet remains the treatment of choice for everyone, especially the elderly.

There has been no end to the proliferation of diet books and new miracle cholesterol-reducing programs. Consumers beware! The latest "revolutionary" program claims that hardening of the arteries can be reversed in a large majority of individuals if they follow a rigid vegetarian diet, and devote approximately 15 to 20 hours of a week to exercise, stress management, and counseling sessions. Obviously, this is a highly impractical program for a vast number of individuals! All of the patients studied had coronary artery disease and x-ray studies demonstrated a decrease in the size of the plaques in the arteries in the study patients. The degree of decrease, however, was small and some experts state that the methods used to detect these changes were not sensitive enough to be relied upon. Confusing the results was the fact that regression or improvement in the artery lesions was also noted in all four women in the *control* group.

The most dramatic difference between the 22 patients in the experimental group and the control group of 19 was the difference in weight changes—a 22-pound loss compared to a 2- to 3-pound gain over a one-year period.

Again, weight loss, which can be accomplished by a sensible low-fat, calorie-restricted diet, coupled with a moderate exercise program, is probably still the key to reducing cardiovascular disease. A program that people can follow within the framework of their daily lives is a must for long-term success. I do not believe that this new "miracle" approach can be followed by more than a few well-to-do individuals who have the time and financial resources and are extremely well intentioned. We must await results of additional trials before accepting the findings of this small study. The public should avoid falling into the trap laid by a massive public relations campaign to sell books or increase the population of a "life-style change" center.

Oat Bran, Garlic, and Other Dietary Substances

There continue to be conflicting data on the value of oat bran to lower blood cholesterol. Many people cannot tolerate the large amounts of this food stuff that is needed to make a difference. Overall, it appears that a high-fiber diet that includes soluble fiber such as that found in oat bran or pysillium (Metamucil) can produce a moderate reduction of cholesterol. However, a large intake of oat bran is not a cure for an elevated cholesterol.

German researchers have recently produced interesting data indicating that the use of garlic may reduce blood cholesterol. In several studies, the herb was given in pill form containing dried garlic powder, and research subjects who took the garlic noted about a 10 percent reduction in serum cholesterol levels. My colleagues and I are presently engaged in a study to confirm this. Garlic is now available in coated tablets such as "Kwai" that apparently do not produce an odor except in a small number of people. Except for the few individuals who develop gastrointestinal symptoms such as diarrhea and cramps in response to garlic, this substance appears to be harmless. If further research confirms that it can lower cholesterol, garlic may well be yet another useful addition to a cholesterol-lowering diet. A small decrease in blood pressure, following the use of garlic, has also been noted in recent studies.

Confusing messages about margarine have appeared in both medical and lay publications following a report from Holland. The investigators reported that certain types of solid margarine contained fatty acids that actually increased serum lipid levels; that the process of producing hard margarine (the kind that is widely used) transforms a low saturated fatty substance into a substance which might be harmful. As with many such studies, the subjects in this investigation were given three to four times the amount of fatty acids than would be obtained from an ordinary U.S. diet that contains margarine. Thus, it is difficult to apply the findings to individuals who use margarine only two to three times a day, on bread, in cooking, etc. I continue to believe that margarine is preferable to butter in a heart-healthy diet, and that we should not abandon or reduce its use on the basis of this study.

More Data on Tobacco Smoke

More data has emerged in the last year confirming the detrimental effects of tobacco smoke. New data also appears to confirm that passive smoke—the smoke inhaled by nonsmokers who are in close proximity to smokers—does have a negative effect. There is evidence that the risk of both lung and heart disease are increased among passive smokers. The risk, however, is not as great as that for smokers. If you don't have any other risk factors for heart or lung disease, passive smoke probably is not going to make much difference. But it may be hazardous to someone who has heart disease or other major risk factors.

In Summary

The remarkable progress in reducing deaths from cardiovascular disease continues. The National Heart, Lung, and Blood Institute has just reported a decrease of over 54 percent in stroke deaths and a more than 45 percent decrease in heart disease deaths in the United States over the past 17 years. This rate of decrease is greater than that achieved in any other industrialized society. In fact, over the same period of time, many Eastern European countries have recorded an increase in deaths from heart disease.

Controlling high blood pressure in more and more people has played a key role in prolonging life and reducing disabilities.

Paying attention to and reducing other risk factors has also paid off. Despite these optimistic statistics, heart and vascular diseases still result in more deaths than any other cause.

As a nation we are on our way toward reducing the burden of heart disease still further. Along the route, we must, however, be wary of the headline producers, the quick fixes, and the miracle programs that might only be suitable for the few, and unaffordable for the majority. The common sense approach to reducing blood pressure and the risk of a stroke or heart attack that was outlined in *Lower Your Blood Pressure and Live Longer* in 1989 has been confirmed by newer data. This approach will work for most people, and without major life-style disruptions, undue expense, or excessive time commitments.